14.95

Karen A. Roberto
Editor

Relationships Between Women in Later Life

Pre-publication
REVIEWS,
COMMENTARIES,
EVALUATIONS . . .

More pre-publication
REVIEWS, COMMENTARIES, EVALUATIONS . . .

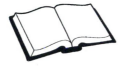

"This book is *a welcome addi- tion to my women's studies and gerontology libraries. The deci- sion to concentrate on relationships between women, rather than on comparisons between men and women is smart and still quite novel. . . .* The authors ask, why should our interest in women's lives and experi- ence only be of concern insofar as how they differ or are similar to men's? Does not the distinctiveness of older women's mutual relation- ships merit attention? These are very good questions.

This book is *well-grounded, theorectically and empirically, but it also goes to the next level and asks, "so what"? The collection of authors shows us ways to apply the information they share, which is certainly a worthwhile endeavor."*

Karen Seccombe, PhD
Associate Professor
Department of Sociology
University of Florida, Gainesville

"Karen A. Roberto's volume . . . is organized into two distinct sections, each addressing the sup- portive qualities of old women's relationships. It begins by examining more traditional types of relation- ships between women: mothers and daughters, grandmothers and grand- daughters, siblings, friends and part- ners, including older lesbians . . . In the second section, the authors explore the supportive functions among sets of older women's rela- tionships that have rarely been ad- dressed in the literature: Catholic sis- ters in later life, female farm opera- tors, older wards and their guardians and women living in retirement communities and nursing homes."

Nancy R. Hooyman, PhD, MSW
Dean
University of Washington
School of Social Work
Seattle

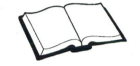

"Roberto's edited volume reflects themes of interconnectedness that have consistently been shown to be primary to the fabric of women's lives. The book is well organized and appropriately divided into two major divisions. The first section provides helpful general information about older women's social relationships across several types including mother/daughter, sibling, grandparent/grandchild, and friend bonds. The second section concentrates on the presentation of information about older women's relationships within specific contexts.

The volume reflects growth in our understanding of older women's social networks and has several strengths. These include the incorporation of results from cross-sectional as well as longitudinal studies; examples of qualitative and quantitative methods; and most importantly, examinations of social bonds across many lifestyles. Chapters reflect the richness of data available when more in-depth studies of women are conducted. Information about rural older women, Catholic sisters, and female farm operators are particularly valuable because they provide insights about the lives of heterogeneous women aging in a variety of situations."

B. Jan McCulloch, PhD
Associate Professor
Department of Family Studies
Sanders-Brown Center on Aging
University of Kentucky

Relationships Between Women in Later Life

Relationships Between Women in Later Life

Karen A. Roberto, PhD
Editor

Relationships Between Women in Later Life, edited by Karen A. Roberto, PhD, was simultaneously issued by The Haworth Press, Inc. under the same title, as a special issue of *Journal of Women & Aging*, Volume 8, Numbers 3/4 1996, J. Dianne Garner, Journal Editor.

Harrington Park Press
An Imprint of
The Haworth Press, Inc.
New York • London

1-56023-091-6

Published by

Harrington Park Press, 10 Alice Street, Binghamton, NY 13904-1580 USA

Harrington Park Press is an imprint of The Haworth Press, Inc., 10 Alice Street, Binghamton, NY 13904-1580 USA.

Relationships Between Women in Later Life has also been published as *Journal of Women & Aging*, Volume 8, Numbers 3/4 1996.

The development, preparation, and publication of this work has been undertaken with great care. However, the publisher, employees, editors, and agents of The Haworth Press and all imprints of The Haworth Press, Inc., including The Haworth Medical Press and Pharmaceutical Products Press, are not responsible for any errors contained herein or for consequences that may ensue from use of materials or information contained in this work. Opinions expressed by the author(s) are not necessarily those of The Haworth Press, Inc.

Library of Congress Cataloging-in-Publication Data

Relationships between women in later life / Karen A. Roberto, editor.
    p. cm.
    "Has also been published as Journal of women & aging, Volume 8, Numbers 3/4, 1996" –T.p. verso.
    Includes bibliographical references (p.) and index.
    ISBN 0-7890-0009-1 (THP : acid-free paper).–ISBN 1-56023-091-6 (HPP : acid-free paper)
    1. Aged women–Social networks. 2. Aged women–Psychology. 3. Interpersonal relations. 4. Intergenerational relations. 5. Female friendship. I. Roberto, Karen A.
HQ1061.R424 1996
306.26–dc20
                                    96-30653
                                        CIP

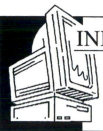

INDEXING & ABSTRACTING

Contributions to this publication are selectively indexed or abstracted in print, electronic, online, or CD-ROM version(s) of the reference tools and information services listed below. This list is current as of the copyright date of this publication. See the end of this section for additional notes.

- *Abstracts in Anthropology*, Baywood Publishing Company, 26 Austin Avenue, P.O. Box 337, Amityville, NY 11701

- *Abstracts in Social Gerontology: Current Literature on Aging*, National Council on the Aging, Library, 409 Third Street SW, 2nd Floor, Washington, DC 20024

- *Abstracts of Research in Pastoral Care & Counseling*, Loyola College, 7135 Minstrel Way, Suite 101, Columbia, MD 21045

- *Academic Index (on-line)*, Information Access Company, 362 Lakeside Drive, Foster City, CA 94404

- *AgeInfo CD-ROM*, Centre for Policy on Ageing, 25-31 Ironmonger Row, London EC1V 4QP, England

- *AgeLine Database*, American Association of Retired Persons, 601 E Street NW, Washington DC 20049

- *Behavioral Medicine Abstracts*, University of Washington, School of Social Work, Seattle, WA 98195

- *Cambridge Scientific Abstracts*, *Risk Abstracts*, Environmental Routenet (accessed via INTERNET), 7200 Wisconsin Avenue #601, Bethesda, MD 20814

- *CNPIEC Reference Guide: Chinese Directory of Foreign Periodicals*, P.O. Box 88, Beijing, People's Republic of China

- *Combined Health Information Database (CHID),* National Institutes of Health, 3 Information Way, Bethesda, MD 20892-3580

- *Current Contents*. . . . see: Institute for Scientific Information

(continued)

- ***Family Studies Database (online and CD/ROM)***, Peters Technology Transfer, 306 East Baltimore Pike, 2nd Floor, Media, PA 19063

- ***Feminist Periodicals: A Current Listing of Contents***, Women's Studies Librarian-at-Large, 728 State Street, 430 Memorial Library, Madison, WI 53706

- ***Guide to Social Science & Religion in Periodical Literature***, National Periodical Library, P.O. Box 3278, Clearwater, FL 34630

- ***Human Resources Abstracts (HRA)***, Sage Publications, Inc., 2455 Teller Road, Newbury Park, CA 91320

- ***IBZ International Bibliography of Periodical Literature***, Zeller Verlag GmbH & Co., P.O.B. 1949, d-49009 Osnabruck, Germany

- ***Index to Periodical Articles Related to Law***, University of Texas, 727 East 26th Street, Austin, TX 78705

- ***Institute for Scientific Information***, 3501 Market Street, Philadelphia, PA 19104. Coverage in:
  b) Research Alerts (current awareness service)
  c) Social SciSearch (magnetic tape)
  d) Current Contents/Social & Behavioral Sciences (weekly current awareness service)

- ***INTERNET ACCESS (& additional networks) Bulletin Board for Libraries ("BUBL"), coverage of information resources on INTERNET, JANET, and other networks.***
  - JANET X.29: UK.AC.BATH.BUBL or 00006012101300
  - TELNET: BUBL.BATH.AC.UK or 138.38.32.45 login 'bubl'
  - Gopher: BUBL.BATH.AC.UK (138.32.32.45). Port 7070
  - World Wide Web: http: / / www.bubl.bath.ac.uk./BUBL/ home.html
  - NISSWAIS: telnetniss.ac.uk (for the NISS gateway)
  The Andersonian Library, Curran Building, 101 St. James Road, Glasgow G4 ONS, Scotland

- ***Master FILE***, EBSCO Publishing, 83 Pine Street, Peabody, MA 01960

(continued)

- *Mental Health Abstracts (online through DIALOG)*, IFI/Plenum Data Company, 3202 Kirkwood Highway, Wilmington, DE 19808

- *National Clearinghouse for Primary Care Information (NCPCI)*, 8201 Greensboro Drive, Suite 600, McLean, VA 22102

- *New Literature on Old Age*, Centre for Policy on Ageing, 25-31 Ironmonger Row, London EC1V 3QP, England

- *Periodical Abstracts, Research II (broad coverage indexing & abstracting data-base from University Microfilms International (UMI) 300 North Zeeb Road, P.O. Box 1346, Ann Arbor, MI 48106-1346)*, UMI Data Courier, P.O. Box 32770, Louisville, KY 40232-2770

- *Periodical Abstracts Select (abstracting & indexing service covering most frequently requested journals in general reference, plus journals requested in libraries serving undergraduate programs, available from University Microfilms International (UMI), 300 North Zeeb Road, P.O. Box 1346, Ann Arbor, MI 48106-1346)*, UMI Data Courier, Attn: Library Services, Box 34660, Louisville, KY 40232

- *SilverPlatter Information, Inc.* **"CD-ROM/online,"** Information Resources Group, P.O. Box 50550, Pasadena, CA 91115-0550

- *Social Planning/Policy & Development Abstracts (SOPODA)*, Sociological Abstracts, Inc., P.O. Box 22206, San Diego, CA 92192-0206

- *Social Science Citation Index* . . . . see: Institute for Scientific Information

- *Social Work Abstracts*, National Association of Social Workers, 750 First Street NW, 8th Floor, Washington, DC 20002

- *Sociological Abstracts (SA)*, Sociological Abstracts, Inc., P.O. Box 22206, San Diego, CA 92192-0206

- *Studies on Women Abstracts*, Carfax Publishing Company, P.O. Box 25, Abingdon, Oxfordshire OX14 3UE, United Kingdom

- *Women Studies Abstracts,* Rush Publishing Company, P.O. Box 1, Rush, NY 14543

- *Women's Studies Index (indexed comprehensively)*, G.K. Hall & Co., 866 Third Avenue, New York, NY 10022

SPECIAL BIBLIOGRAPHIC NOTES

related to special journal issues (separates)
and indexing/abstracting

☐ indexing/abstracting services in this list will also cover material in any "separate" that is co-published simultaneously with Haworth's special thematic journal issue or DocuSerial. Indexing/abstracting usually covers material at the article/chapter level.

☐ monographic co-editions are intended for either non-subscribers or libraries which intend to purchase a second copy for their circulating collections.

☐ monographic co-editions are reported to all jobbers/wholesalers/approval plans. The source journal is listed as the "series" to assist the prevention of duplicate purchasing in the same manner utilized for books-in-series.

☐ to facilitate user/access services all indexing/abstracting services are encouraged to utilize the co-indexing entry note indicated at the bottom of the first page of each article/chapter/contribution.

☐ this is intended to assist a library user of any reference tool (whether print, electronic, online, or CD-ROM) to locate the monographic version if the library has purchased this version but not a subscription to the source journal.

☐ individual articles/chapters in any Haworth publication are also available through the Haworth Document Delivery Services (HDDS).

CONTENTS

ABOUT THE EDITOR

Karen A. Roberto, PhD, is Director of the Center for Gerontology at Virginia Polytechnic Institute and State University in Blacksburg. She is the former Coordinator of the Gerontology Program at the University of North Carolina in Greeley. Editor of the books "The Elderly Caregiver" (Sage, 1993) and "Older Women with Chronic Pain" (The Haworth Press, Inc., 1994), Dr. Roberto is the author of numerous journal articles and book chapters addressing family and friend relationships in later life and the psychosocial issues facing older women with osteoporosis. She is a Fellow of the Gerontological Society of America and the Book Review Editor for the *Journal of Women & Aging.*

Preface

I am . . .
Derived from family
Embedded in community
Not isolated from prevailing values
Though having unique experiences
In certain roles and status . . .

–Ruth Harriet Jacobs (1991, p. 37)

Relationships with others are at the core of our existence. Throughout the life cycle, involvement within our social networks helps shape every aspect of our lives. The family serves as the basis for the structure and development of personal relationships. From this foundation, we build other types of informal and formal alliances.

This volume examines several different types of relationships between women in later life. The contributing authors employ a variety of quantitative and qualitative methodologies to provide readers with insights into the multifaceted nature of older women's relationships. They use several different frameworks to advance theoretical understanding and practical knowledge of both informal and formal connections. The older women studied present a broad spectrum of life and social circumstances that influenced the development and maintenance of their personal relationships.

The decision to concentrate on relationships between women, rather than taking a more global approach to the study of relationships that would have included women's relationships with men or gender comparisons,

---

[Haworth co-indexing entry note]: "Preface." Roberto, Karen A. Co-published simultaneously in the *Journal of Women & Aging* (The Haworth Press, Inc.) Vol. 8, Nos. 3/4, 1996, pp. 1-4; and: *Relationships Between Women in Later Life* (ed: Karen A. Roberto) The Haworth Press, Inc., 1996, pp. 1-4; and: *Relationships Between Women in Later Life* (ed: Karen A. Roberto) Harrington Park Press, an imprint of The Haworth Press, Inc., 1996, pp. 1-4. [Single or multiple copies of this article are available from the Haworth Document Delivery Service: 1-800-342-9678, 9:00 a.m. - 5:00 p.m. (EST). E-mail address: getinfo@haworth.com]

1

resulted for a variety of reasons. First, women are the fastest growing segment of the older population. Their sheer numbers and the unique health, personal, and social issues they face make aging largely a woman's issue. Second, society often views relationships as primarily a woman's domain. Much of the recent research on women's relationships in later life has focused on women as caregivers, a role in which they predominate. Researchers have paid less attention to the other types of relationships in which older women are involved. Finally, it is widely accepted that the interpersonal relationships of women and men differ. Significant bonds form between women throughout the life cycle. This is not to say that the connections between older women and men and between men in later life are of any less importance, but only that the distinctiveness of older women's mutual relationships deserves special attention.

I organized this collection of papers into two distinct but overlapping sections. The authors of the first set of papers examine long-term, more traditional types of relationships between women: mothers and daughters, grandmothers and granddaughters, siblings, friends and partners. The authors further our understanding of these informal relationships by examining unique aspects and/or circumstances influencing the bond between the women. Rosemary Blieszner, Paula Usita, and Jay Mancini employ gerontological and feminist frameworks in their investigation of late-life mother-daughter relationships. They discovered that close mother-daughter relationships result from satisfying interactions, have a history of little conflict, involve few control issues, and encompass many opportunities for informal, non-obligatory contact. Using the revised theory of intergenerational solidarity as her conceptual framework, Vira Kivett examines the salience of the grandmother-granddaughter tie when older women migrate. She found that associational solidarity was primarily a function of the opportunity structure proximity and, to a smaller extent, the age of the granddaughter. Jean Pearson Scott presents findings from a longitudinal investigation of the structural and contact features of sibling relationships. She discovered that although there was a "thinning" of the sibling network in late old age, siblings continue to play an active role in the kin networks of rural older women. I examine the interactions of older women and multiple members of their close friend network. The responses of the women revealed that within their network of close friends, they have a "preferred" friend with whom they interact socially and frequently turn to for intimacy and understanding. Dena Shenk and Elise Fullmer focus on the interactive nature of the relationship between personal and public constructions of lesbianism in the lives of older women. They present a case study of a lesbian in her 80s living in a small rural town that illustrates how she developed and maintained her relationship with her partner despite societal and cultural constraints.

In the second section, the authors focus their attention on the supportive functions of older women's relationships. They explore the informal and more formal relationships of various sub-groups of women in their later years: women with a formal religious affiliation, female farm operators, care-recipients, and women living in structured environments (i.e., CCRCs and nursing homes). Joyce Mercier, Mack Shelley II, and Edward Powers examine the influence of social relationships on the self-esteem of Catholic sisters in later life. They report that for these religious women, having close friends, having relationships with children, being active socially in various groups, and interacting with their families are very rewarding and positively related to self-esteem. M. Jean Turner investigates the acceptability of potential in-home and live-in social support options available for middle-aged and older female farm operators. Overall, these women showed resistance to help except from a spouse, emphasizing their strong desire to remain independent. Enid Opal Cox and Ruth Parsons present the experiences of elderly women care-recipients participating in an empowerment-oriented group and the impact of this participation on their interpersonal relationships. They report that group activities (e.g., promoting a sense of reciprocity and mutual respect) had a positive influence on the establishment and maintenance of the women's relationships, both within and outside the group. Robbyn Wacker and Pat Keith explore the relationship between older women and their female guardians. They found that the formal relationship between the women influenced the guardians' feelings toward the wards and shaped the guardians' perceptions of aging and the conceptions of their own aging. Margaret Perkinson and David Rockemann investigate the formation of friendships by women who recently moved to a new retirement community. They discovered that the women's marital status was a major factor in the selection of friends within this setting. Bethel Ann Powers describes the relationships among older women living in a nursing home. She suggests that the women set limits in their relationships and warded off negative interactions by resisting and evading relationships beyond their tolerance.

This volume brings forth new knowledge and understanding of relationships between women in later life. Not only did the older women who participated in the various studies shape their relationships, but their relationships actively shaped their lives. As the editor of this volume, it is my hope that practitioners will consider what we have learned about the importance of personal relationships between older women and incorporate it into their daily work. In addition, I encourage researchers, from a variety of disciplines, to act on the authors' suggestions for future work and continue to build upon the findings presented.

I would like to thank the authors for their hard work and dedication. Their commitment to the study of older women and late life relationships in general, and to this project in particular, made editing an enjoyable process. I would also like to thank three of my former graduate students at the University of Northern Colorado, Flora Robinson, Connie Seay and Michael Skoglund who helped me with the tedious tasks of proofreading and referencing.

Karen A. Roberto, PhD

REFERENCE

Jacobs, R. H. (1991). *Be an outrageous older woman—a R*A*S*P: Remarkable aging smart person.* Manchester, CT: Knowledge, Ideas, & Trends.

PART I:
PRIMARY RELATIONSHIPS

Diversity and Dynamics in Late-Life Mother-Daughter Relationships

Rosemary Blieszner, PhD
Paula M. Usita, MS
Jay A. Mancini, PhD

SUMMARY. We employed gerontological and feminist frameworks in an investigation of normative late-life mother-daughter relation-

Rosemary Blieszner is Professor, Paula M. Usita is a Doctoral Candidate, and Jay A. Mancini is Professor, all at the Department of Family and Child Development, Virginia Polytechnic Institute and State University, Blacksburg, VA 24061-0416.

The data used in this study are from *Family Interaction and Psychological Well-Being: An Analysis of Older Parent-Adult Child Relationships,* research sponsored by the AARP Andrus Foundation and the Virginia Tech Educational Foundation; Jay A. Mancini, Principal Investigator.

[Haworth co-indexing entry note]: "Diversity and Dynamics in Late-Life Mother-Daughter Relationships." Blieszner, Rosemary, Paula M. Usita, and Jay A. Mancini. Co-published simultaneously in the *Journal of Women & Aging* (The Haworth Press, Inc.) Vol. 8, Nos. 3/4, 1996, pp. 5-24; and: *Relationships Between Women in Later Life* (ed: Karen A. Roberto) The Haworth Press, Inc., 1996, pp. 5-24; and: *Relationships Between Women in Later Life* (ed: Karen A. Roberto) Harrington Park Press, an imprint of The Haworth Press, Inc., 1996, pp. 5-24. [Single or multiple copies of this article are available from the Haworth Document Delivery Service: 1-800-342-9678, 9:00 a.m. - 5:00 p.m. (EST). E-mail address: getinfo@haworth.com]

ships. Building on previous research, we used data from a representative sample of older mothers to explore in depth the predictors of relationship quality and the satisfactions and complaints prevalent in relationships with mothers in later life. Structured interview data revealed that the intimacy dimension of relationship quality is influenced by contact satisfaction, past conflict, control issues, and amount of discretionary contact whereas the antagonism dimension is affected by present conflict, control issues, and mother's education. Analysis of semistructured interview data showed that elements of companionship, cohesion, and conflict underscore perceptions of relationship quality. The discussion and conclusion locate the findings within the gerontology-feminist literature and provide implications for researchers and practitioners. *[Article copies available from The Haworth Document Delivery Service: 1-800-342-9678. E-mail address: getinfo@haworth.com]*

Gerontology and feminism share common goals: development of social consciousness about the inequities confronting older people and women, utilization of theories and methods that accurately depict the everyday life experiences of older people and women, and promotion of change in the conditions of older people and women (Reinharz, 1986; Walker & Thompson, 1984). Gerontologists employing feminist approaches commit themselves to understanding and improving older women's lives.

In this paper, we acknowledge the intersection of gerontological and feminist frameworks as we explore normative late-life mother-daughter relationships. We believe this project contributes to a better understanding of women's lives because of several key features of the research. First, we focus on a relationship that is long-enduring and very meaningful to many women. Second, we give attention to typical associations, as opposed to nonnormative ones, to avoid problematizing the mother-daughter relationship (Allen & Walker, 1992). Third, we incorporate quantitative and qualitative methods of inquiry to highlight multiple dimensions of mother-daughter relationships. Fourth, our findings have application for professionals in gerontology and family arenas who seek to improve the quality of women's lives and relationships.

We begin with an overview of previous research that focused specifically on adult mother-daughter relationships. Building on those findings, we use data from a representative sample of older adults to explore in greater depth the predictors of relationship quality and the satisfactions and complaints prevalent in relationships when mothers are elderly. Our discussion locates the findings within the gerontology-feminist literature and spells out some implications for researchers and practitioners.

BACKGROUND

The gerontological literature on mother-daughter relationships recognizes that this long-enduring affiliation has the potential of influencing adult development in significant ways (Henwood & Coughlan, 1993; Troll, 1987). Previously investigated topics include (a) implications for relationship quality of affection and support provision and of multiple roles, (b) perceptions of psychological closeness, and (c) care provision.

Affection and Support

One interesting focus of the literature on elderly mother-adult daughter relationships has been the extent to which each partner's affection and support needs were met and subsequent implications for relationship quality. In a study of aid patterns and attachment, Thompson and Walker (1984) found that mothers were more attached to their daughters than daughters were to their mothers. Further, reciprocity in the exchange of assistance mediated feelings of attachment in both mothers and daughters. When reciprocity was high, both mothers and daughters reported high levels of emotional attachment (Thompson & Walker, 1984). Bromberg (1983) reported that patterns of mutual aid between mothers and daughters were unaffected by any fluctuations in the quality of the relationship. Older mothers stated that they received affective and instrumental aid from their daughters while they also provided affective aid to their daughters (Bromberg, 1983). Walker and Thompson (1983), however, cautioned researchers against assuming that frequency of contact and support provision directly signify the quality of the relationship. Those variables accounted for only 11% of the variance in mother-daughter intimacy in their study. Rather, they advocated assessing more detailed information about the nature of the interactions that take place during visiting and helping.

Multiple Roles

Walker and Thompson's (1983) recommendation was important because it acknowledged that visiting and helping could occur under either discretionary or strained circumstances. Researchers have examined the late-life mother-daughter relationship within the context of pertinent structural variables such as role status. Inquiry into the influence of competing role statuses, or role strains, on relationship involvement and relationship quality resulted in mixed findings. In a study of mothers' and daughters' marriage, employment, and parenthood statuses, Walker, Thompson, and

Morgan (1987) found that neither role position nor combinations of roles influenced the level of interdependence between mothers and daughters. Scharlach (1987) also reported that daughters' role participation did not interfere with the provision of support or with relationship quality. Baruch and Barnett (1983), however, found the opposite. Daughters who were themselves mothers or were single described their relationships with their mothers as less rewarding than daughters who were not mothers or were married. Their findings also contrast with Fischer's (1981, 1986) observation that daughters who were themselves mothers viewed their relationships with their mothers positively.

Psychological Closeness

Most of the research on normative mother-daughter relationships is grounded in psychodynamic or social learning models. Psychodynamic models focus on attachment, instinctual, and bonding issues between mothers and daughters, whereas social learning models focus on the principle sources of reinforcement that teach daughters to behave similarly to their mothers (Boyd, 1989; Cohler, 1988; Henwood & Coughlan, 1993; Weitzman, 1984). These theoretical perspectives problematically confine mother-daughter relationships to prescribed explanations that do not empower women nor allow them to describe how they actively shape their lives.

Recent research on adult mothers and daughters highlights diversity by taking a perspective that questions the presumed inherent closeness in mother-daughter relationships. Through discourse analysis, Henwood (1993) discovered that although themes of mother-daughter closeness emerged, issues of difficulty and dissatisfaction also surfaced. Similarly, O'Connor (1990) reported that daughters did not necessarily describe their relationships with their mothers as very close. Contrary to the accepted belief that mothers and daughters are always close, which sentimentalizes the relationship (Allen & Walker, 1992), these studies convey a broader picture of interaction patterns and feelings.

Care Provision

Consequent to the emphasis on psychoanalytic and social learning perspectives, researchers examine the mother-daughter relationship in the context of providing care. Restricting research to the issues of caregiving obscures the range of possible exchanges between mothers and daughters. This is particularly true when the focus is on the burdensome aspects of helping, with little or no attention paid to the benefits gained from doing so or the contributions of the care recipient to the relationship (Allen & Walker, 1992; Barnett, 1988). Assumptions about the hardships of caregiving and the passive stance of care recipients restrict the understanding of women's interpretation of the caregiving experience. Additionally, an exclusive focus on caregiving distracts attention from normative mother-daughter relationships (O'Connor, 1990).

An Expanded Research Paradigm

The findings mentioned here illustrate the range of adult mother-daughter relationship functions and influences on them. Previous research reveals that it is not sufficient to focus exclusively on nurturant and affectionate aspects of interaction. Neither is it appropriate to assume that conflict overruns mother-daughter relationships. Assistance is bidirectional, not unidirectional. Thus, recognition of the multifaceted nature of the relationship evidences advancement over the previous research paradigms that either problematized or sentimentalized it (Allen & Walker, 1992). In place of confining perceptions of caregiving to negativity and the mother-daughter relationship itself to either affectionate or problematic domains, there needs to be a more comprehensive approach to the examination of women's relational ideas. Essential is a concerted effort to examine the strengths of mother-daughter relationships, especially from the perspective of older mothers, who have been studied less often than younger mothers (Bromberg, 1987; Troll, 1988). Thus, our investigation targeted a full range of interaction variables, first, by specifically inquiring about both beneficial and undesirable aspects, and second, by allowing elderly mothers to express assessments of their relationships with daughters in their own words.

METHOD

Procedure

Sample. Data were collected in 1984 and 1985. A modified probability sampling design was used to derive a target sample of 500 people from the population aged 65 years or older (13% of the total; U.S. Bureau of the Census, 1982) within the urbanized area of Roanoke, Virginia. Census data were employed to segment Roanoke according to year-round dwellings. The segments were grouped into 10 zones and 6 sampling units were randomly selected within each zone. Interviewers canvassed all dwelling units within these sampling units and asked all residents who met the age and parental requirements to participate in the interview. Of the 635 potential interviewees, 494 of them (78%) comprised the original sample. The sample characteristics compared favorably with both local and national census data regarding race, marital status, sex, and education (Mancini & Blieszner, 1993). The main difference was that all respondents in this study had living children, whereas about 20% of people 65 and older in the general population have no living children.

Of the 494 participants, 196 (40%) were mothers who reported on a relationship with an adult daughter; we analyzed this subset of the data in the present paper. The average age of the mothers was 73, with a range of 61 to 97 years and a median of 71 years. Eighty-two percent were White. They had resided in their neighborhoods an average of 22 years; 40% lived by themselves. When interviewed, 38% were married (M years = 45) and 55% were widowed (M years = 14). Although only 6% were employed at the time of the interview, 66% had been employed at age 50. The mothers averaged 10 years of formal education with 21% reporting more than 12 years of schooling. The average number of living children was just under three; 26% had only one living child.

The daughters about whom the mothers spoke ranged in age from 22 to 74 years, with a mean and median age of 45 years. Most of the daughters were married (68%). They had an average of 2.2 children and the majority enjoyed good to excellent health (76%). Two-thirds of the daughters lived in the same city as the mothers, 12% lived within 100 miles of the area, and 13% lived within 500 miles. Only 8% of the daughters lived farther than 500 miles from their mothers.

From the pool of 494 respondents, a subsample of 52 women and men was drawn by simple random selection for semistructured follow-up interviews conducted four to six months later. The response rate for the second interview was 90% and the respondents represented the larger group from which they were selected. The subsample included 21 fathers and 31 mothers. Data from the 15 mothers who discussed relationships with daughters provide the basis of the qualitative analyses presented in this paper. These mothers averaged 72 years of age (Range = 66 to 85 years). Most of them were widowed (N = 11), a few were married (N = 3), and one was divorced. Most were White (N = 10), four women were Black, and the race of one woman is unknown.

Interviews. Trained interviewers interviewed respondents in their own homes or apartments. Those who had more than one child reported on their relationship with either the child to whom they felt the closest (17%

of the 196 mothers who reported on daughters) or, if unwilling to select on that basis, the child with whom they had the most contact (52% of the 196 mothers who reported on daughters; the selection basis for 31% of these mothers is unknown). The same child was the focus of both interviews for those in the follow-up subsample. The initial interviews had a mean length of one hour. The follow-up sessions lasted one and a half to two hours on average.

The structured interviews included 11 indicators of relationship interaction and quality and 9 indicators of parent and child demographic characteristics. The relationship items tapped intimacy (e.g., trust, understanding); antagonism (e.g., sarcasm, irritating tone); family involvement (in each other's lives); frequency of task, companionate, discretionary, and obligatory contact (e.g., "How often do you see/talk on the phone with [daughter] . . . because one of you needs help from the other? . . . just to talk, share experiences and enjoy each other's company? . . . because you really want to? . . . because you think you should?"); satisfaction with contact; past and present conflict; and difficulty with making decisions (relationship control issues) (Mancini & Blieszner, 1993).

The follow-up interviews began with a general question about the mother's relationship with her daughter: "I would like you to talk about your present relationship with [daughter]. Perhaps the easiest way for you to begin would be to discuss the first things that come to mind when you think about [daughter]." If the respondents required probing, the interviewers asked other questions designed to parallel the topics addressed in the structured interview.

Data Analysis

We analyzed the structured interview data via product-moment correlations and stepwise multiple regression procedures. These statistical procedures provide a multivariate assessment of the components of relationship quality across the large pool of respondents (cf. Acock & Schumm, 1993).

Two research assistants listened to the tapes of the semistructured interviews, transcribed relevant passages verbatim, and coded the responses according to the relationship dimensions expressed by the respondents. Two of the authors then reviewed the transcriptions several times, added more detailed coding, and identified and revised categories and themes emerging from the data (Taylor & Bogdan, 1984). This process allows the actual comments of the respondents to guide the search for and interpretation of theoretical meanings in the data (Rosenblatt & Fischer, 1993). The qualitative data thus complements the quantitative ones by providing extensive detail as to perceptions of influences on relationship quality.

FINDINGS

Predictors of Relationship Quality

We assessed diverse aspects of relationship quality by exploring a positive and a negative dimension within the structured interview data. The positive indicator was intimacy and the negative one was antagonism. The results of the regression analyses revealed that greater intimacy in the mother-daughter relationship was associated with more satisfaction with contacts ($\beta = .17$), less past conflict ($\beta = -.29$), less difficulty in decision-making ($\beta = -.29$), and more discretionary contact ($\beta = .17$). In contrast, higher antagonism was related to more present conflict ($\beta = .30$), more difficulty in decision-making ($\beta = .30$), and lower parental education ($\beta = -.16$) (All variables significant at $p < .001$; $R^2 = .31$ for intimacy and .28 for antagonism).

Further Exploration of Relationship Quality

We used the results of the qualitative data analysis procedures to gain insight into the relationship dynamics that contribute to the associations revealed by the regression analyses. Three major dimensions of mother-daughter relationship dynamics that appeared to affect relationship quality emerged from the semistructured interview data (see Table 1). The first was *companionship,* involving descriptions of mother-daughter communication and interaction patterns. The second was *cohesion,* or feelings of closeness and togetherness between the mothers and daughters. The third dynamic was *conflict,* concerning the extent of and reactions to disagreements between mothers and daughters.

Companionship. The 15 mothers reported a variety of forms of contact and assistance exchanged with their daughters. They revealed both balanced and unbalanced exchanges, reflecting responsiveness to the particular life circumstances and needs of the mothers and daughters. For example, the mothers who were in poor health relied heavily on their daughters for various forms of aid. In one case, the mother had recently suffered a stroke and her daughter did all household tasks and provided necessary transportation:

TABLE 1. Dimensions of Relationship Quality

Category	Dimensions
Companionship	Responsiveness to Life Circumstances and Needs
	Exchanges of Assistance, balanced and unbalanced
	Communication, frequency and quality
Cohesion	Closeness and Togetherness
	Interdependence, Independence, Dependence
	Loyalty and Thoughtfulness
Conflict	Minimal, little effect on relationship
	Avoidance Tactics
	Circumstantial Causes
	Serious, detrimental to relationship

> I think of [daughter] as someone to take care of me. She has been living here with me. She fixes my meals and gets my medicine and sees that I'm taken care of. She does everything you would in your own home . . . I don't want for anything. [Daughter] and her husband are good to me. They take me wherever I need to go. They take me to the doctor and they take me to church.

But even in the absence of serious illness, some mothers deemed their daughters as giving them more help than they gave the daughters:

> She's been awfully good to me, in every way, when I'm sick and when I'm well, when I'm in a good humor and when I'm in a bad humor. She furnishes me a place to live and she furnishes me food.

> I don't know what I'd do without her. I enjoy having her [live] right across the street . . . We shop together and work some in the yard together. Since I lost my husband, I don't know what I'd do if I didn't have her. In some ways I give to her, but I don't know if I give as much to her as she gives to me.

Other mothers, though, find they must continue to support their daughters as they did when the daughters were young. For example, one mother discussed a daughter who had been married four times and had a history of psychiatric problems:

> I raised the oldest two children until they were eight and nine years old . . . About the only time she calls me [is when] she wants something. She wants money or she wants to use my phone to call her daughter in Texas or one of the children needs something. If she wants [something] I get it for her. But I don't approve of it. She has never been one who could accept responsibility . . . I have always done more for her than she has done for me.

Even in less problematic circumstances, some mothers reported giving more to their daughters than they received:

> We do have an unusual relationship. She had four small children within five years. She was really confined to home and of course I helped her. I helped her quite a bit. I helped her with the children. I tried to give her all the help I could. We just grew close that way. Of course, we were always close.

> Well, sometimes I give more [to the relationship] than [daughter] does, like advice.

The descriptions of balanced exchanges reflect still another pattern of helping. In general, the mothers described these relationships as warm and close:

> [Daughter] is all I have . . . I think we go very well together. I couldn't do without her and I don't think she could do without me.

Speaking about her daughter who is divorced and works in nursing, a mother reported:

> She's always willing to do what she can, [for example] give me advice about a doctor . . . [We] help her out 'cause she was left alone with four boys. We done everything to help her out and help the boys.

During another interview, the daughter sat in the background, confirming the mother's assertions about providing extensive child care at no cost. The mother said:

> She thinks she's as nice to me as I am to her. I think I give more . . . I don't have a car. If I want to go somewhere and she's not working, she'll take me. If I need something and she got [it], I can get it. She washes for me.

Thus, although the mother's provision of child care to her daughter was quite prominent in her assessment, she did acknowledge several ways in which her daughter reciprocated with valuable help.

Another aspect of companionship is communication. For the most part, the mothers' narratives reflected frequent, open communication that enhanced feelings of closeness. This example depicts the mother's evaluation of her daughter's openness:

> She tells a person how she feels. She don't beat around the bush. Anything she wants you to know she goes right ahead and tells you. Even with me.

Several mothers commented, with apparent pleasure, on how often their daughters contacted them:

> We talk each morning.

> I talk with her two or three times a day. If she's too busy during the day, she always call me at night.

> And when [daughter] and them's gone during the winter, she calls me. She calls me about once a month, she calls all of us about once a month.

These interview segments further illustrate the value of communication to the mothers:

> I love to hear her opinions, so she'll give me her opinions. Then she'll say, "Now you're going to have to think that over for yourself, Mother."

> She always asks me, "How are you feeling this morning?" She keeps me up [happy].

On the other hand, in difficult relationships, communication is less frequent and less beneficial to relationship quality:

> She has quite a hot temper. She will storm back at me. Generally, we can talk. Of course, I'm very critical because I don't approve of a lot of things [that she does].

> We don't share much together. I don't tell her nothing. We don't discuss feelings.

These insights into companionship suggest that although many mothers and daughters enjoy each other's company, spend as much time as possible together, and have meaningful communication, the excessive needs and difficulties of the mother or daughter put a strain on their relationships. These aspects of companionship also affect feelings of cohesion within the relationship.

Cohesion. Reflected in comments that indicate interdependence, independence, and dependence in the relationships is the importance of closeness and togetherness to both mothers and daughters. The following quotation incorporates both interdependence and independence:

> We go for lunch. We go shopping . . . I may go three or four days or a week and not see her, but we talk. I feel like that starts my day. We just go on. I have my friends . . . I try not to interfere with her life. She and her husband go and do things together. Sometimes we go out with them.

Interdependence between this mother and daughter revolves around concern for safety:

> They [friends] know that we're very close. We're together so much, for one thing. Whenever she goes out of town, I go with her if possible and whenever I have to go out of town, she goes with me. She doesn't like for me to drive alone and I don't like for her to drive alone.

In contrast, this segment illustrates cohesion in the context of dependence on the mother's part:

> I was telling [daughter] that I would rather go in a nursing home than to bother them. She said not as long as she lived she wouldn't let me go in a nursing home. So, you couldn't ask for nothing more than that I wouldn't think.

Loyalty and thoughtfulness are also important aspects of cohesion:

> She helped me out with my problems. If things don't go right, she stands by her mother.

> If I wasn't feeling good, I'd tell her. But then, she don't take too much for granted. At my age, she don't know what to expect.

> She's very thoughtful. She thinks about us. [If] she goes away, gone overnight or something, they always call. We know where they are. She's just very thoughtful.

From these descriptions comes a sense of the importance to mothers of feeling close to their daughters and of their daughters displaying such closeness through words and actions. The mothers clearly value and appreciate the sense of togetherness that seems to prevail in most of these normative relationships. Nevertheless, sometimes difficulties did arise.

Conflict. We probed specifically for evidence of conflict in the relationships because researchers often ignore negative aspects of close relationships. Some mothers in our subsample denied that they ever had any disagreements with their daughters. Others claimed they never argued with their daughters yet did report examples of conflicts. Only a few mothers indicated extensive conflict, usually in the context of the daughters' problems. Typical of the remarks from the group who reported no conflicts were these:

> I can reason with [daughter] and she understands. We just sit down and talk it over. We never have an argument. Not that we're perfect, but it's just not necessary.

> A lot of people, if they can find the least little thing, they just build it up and build it up. But we don't do that.

Among the mothers who believed that their disagreements were minor and had no serious effects on their relationships, most mentioned that they actively sought to prevent arguments. These types of comments were common:

> We haven't had an argument since she has been here. Sometimes she may say things that don't sit so well with me. And, I know there are plenty of times that I say things that she don't like. But we don't have what you would call arguments. I can't think of arguments that we have really had about our relationship. [We] avoid them.

> We don't disagree very much. I don't bother. She's an old lady now and knows her own business. I don't interfere at all.

[If we ever disagree about things], I just keep it to myself.

That's something we don't do [argue]. She says I'm always telling her but I think that I've got to the age that I don't pay any attention. They're always telling me what to do and I've got to the age where I don't say anything, I just let it go and go on and do what I want to do.

Some mothers who admitted to arguing with their daughters negated the seriousness of any discord:

I just say words. It's not going to be horrible. I laugh at [daughter]. I don't pay any attention to [daughter].

Everybody comes to our house mostly says how good we get along together. A lot of parents say they couldn't live with their children . . . Of course, we have our arguments. Everybody has their ups and downs.

The consequences were not serious because the mothers recognized that their daughters were looking out for the mothers' best interests:

I guess we argue a little bit, not a great deal though . . . She tries to get me out more . . . I guess I'm a little lazy.

She's always on to me . . . I fix birthday dinners and during the holidays I do right much cooking and [daughter], she's always onto me about [that] because then the next day I don't get up. I have to stay in bed because I can't walk then the next day . . . And she's always fussing to me about it.

Another rather benign form of conflict occurred because of circumstances, in this case a temporarily shared residence, rather than because of problems in the relationship per se:

We get along fine. We get along better since she's been in her own place. When we were here together we had problems. This house is too small for two, you know. Everybody got on everybody's nerves.

In contrast to the previous examples, the following comments typify the most serious conflict described by the mothers. Both examples involve relationships in which the daughters have numerous personal problems and, from the mothers' point of view, are not carrying out their responsibilities properly (e.g., holding down a job and taking appropriate care of their children):

> She has always been a big problem to us. We haven't had too many arguments lately because I don't say too much to upset her. It's usually about neglecting her children. Rarely will she tell me the truth and tell me if anything is wrong.

> She knows I'm right so she don't have too much to say. She just listens because she knows if I really get mad with her then I wouldn't keep her daughter, so she lays low.

These normative mother-daughter relationships are not entirely free from strife, but most mothers consider any conflict to be minor and report few serious implications of it. Instead, they convey the impression that they have the ability to avoid major conflict, expect to have routine disagreements, and can easily handle any discordant issues in their interactions with their daughters.

DISCUSSION

We highlighted mother-daughter bonds to give attention, using a broad array of variables, to the longest-lived parent-child relationship—one that has been interpreted by some previous analysts within restrictive conceptual and methodological frameworks. The mothers participating in this research were community residents in relatively good health who did not require extensive help from their daughters. Thus, the results offset the impression of problematized relationships that occurs when researchers focus only on the burdens of caregiving.

Taken together, the quantitative and qualitative findings complement each other and provide a more complete view of interaction dynamics within normative adult mother-daughter relationships than previously available. As revealed in the regression analyses, close mother-daughter relationships in adulthood are likely to include satisfying interactions, have a history of little conflict, involve few control issues, and encompass many opportunities for informal, non-obligatory contact. In contrast, conflict and control issues characterize antagonistic mother-daughter relationships. Probing deeper into mother-daughter affiliations via the qualitative data revealed that relationship quality hinges on evidence of companionship, cohesion, and fairly trivial conflict.

The companionship patterns reflected diversity of interaction and communication according to the needs and abilities of the mothers and daughters. In some cases, the mothers assisted their daughters more than the daughters helped them. Other cases showed the reverse pattern and still others encompassed balanced exchanges. For the most part, communication was open and direct and it enhanced the mothers' positive feelings about their relationships. The more troubled relationships tended to include less discussion of feelings and less effective communication. Most of the mothers provided numerous illustrations of cohesion in their relationships with their daughters, reporting on perceptions of closeness and togetherness from multiple perspectives such as interdependence and loyalty. Sometimes conflict occurred in these high-quality relationships, but it did not seem to diminish their cohesion. Relationships in which the daughters had serious personal problems, in contrast, appeared fraught with dissension along with other negative elements.

These findings extend the research on late-life mother-daughter relationships mentioned previously. Consonant with Bromberg (1983) and Thompson and Walker (1984), we found evidence of affection and support that appeared to continue regardless of minor fluctuations in getting along. Similar to Henwood (1993) and O'Connor (1990), we discovered that interaction dynamics are not all positive or all negative, but typically include some dissatisfactions along with the pleasures. The comments from the mothers about their relationships with their daughters illustrate the complexities and ambiguities within this relationship upon which Troll (1987) speculated and answered some of the questions she raised. We learned, for example, that the troubled mother-daughter relationships had been that way for a long time and probably did not become so merely because the mothers were elders and the daughters were adults. We also observed that the relationships are fluid and usually the mothers and daughters accommodate the fluctuations. That is, shifts among interdependence, independence, and dependence seem to occur naturally, according to each partner's needs, and do not appear to interfere greatly with overall relationship quality.

In summary, relationships between elderly mothers and their daughters when mothers are living independently in the community and daughters are providing companionship, but not day-to-day care, reflect generally positive interaction patterns. Not all such relationships are positive, however, particularly when daughters have long-standing personal problems. Findings for companionship, cohesion, and conflict underscore the multidimensional character of these constructs and suggest several research and practice implications.

IMPLICATIONS

Feminist researchers are challenged to demonstrate how their findings can improve the lives of women (Thompson, 1992; Walker & Thompson, 1984). Toward that end, we offer some recommendations for researchers, educators, and gerontological practitioners who strive to assist women in the discovery and utilization of their strengths.

Research. At an indirect level of application, the findings from this investigation suggest that future research on adult mother-daughter relationships—or other family relationships in adulthood, for that matter—should foster the emergence of diverse points of view. According to our findings, women and their relationships are heterogeneous, with many unique features evident within particular dyads (cf. Walker & Thompson, 1984). Researchers should strive to discover other untapped domains of experience.

Besides strengthening the focus on women's experiences and relationships, future researchers must give attention to issues of racial, ethnic, and class group membership as they affect relationships. Although our analysis elaborates diversity regarding relationship dimensions, our sample did not permit separate examination of the effects of structural variables on mother-daughter relationships. Through acknowledging and accepting the variety of life experiences of both mothers and daughters, and how those circumstances shape the mother-daughter relationship, women's experiences become a source and justification of knowledge. This approach is consistent with the goals espoused by both feminist family scholars (Thompson, 1992) and feminist gerontologists (Hendricks, 1993).

One way to open the door to the diversity of experiences in adult relationships is to utilize a combination of research methods with a given sample. As we have shown in this paper, use of qualitative methods to explore intensively the findings reached through quantitative analysis has beneficial outcomes. Quantitative analyses identified the interaction variables relevant to two dimensions of relationship quality and qualitative inquiry allowed more detailed explanations of those variables to emerge. For example, we elaborated on the results for conflict from the structured interviews by uncovering stories in the semistructured interviews about minor, easily handled disagreements in most relationships along with more serious, pervasive arguments in relationships with daughters who were failing to live up to the mothers' expectations.

Intervention. At a direct intervention level, one use of the research results would be in discussion and support groups for mothers and daughters. The purpose of such groups is to assist the participants in identifying their concerns and finding solutions for them. For example, Bromberg

(1987) reported on the benefits of a group comprising mothers and their daughters, who met for eight sessions to discuss the effects they had on each other's aging and the expectations each held for their relationship. These women explored the transition from a power-based relationship when the daughters were children to a mature, renegotiated sharing between peers. They discovered mutual concerns and affirmed their interdependence.

Similarly, group leaders and community educators can use our research results to acquaint participants with a wide range of responses to mother-daughter interactions. For example, they could encourage group members to acknowledge mutual help between mothers and daughters, to strive for open communication, and to seek activities they can enjoy together. Further, professionals can use our findings to reassure mother-daughter pairs about their normalcy and their commonalities with other women experiencing similar issues. Becoming aware of the multifaceted dynamics within a myriad of aspects of the relationship, as evidenced by the present study participants, might stimulate other mother-daughter pairs to identify and appreciate multiple dimensions of their own relational strengths. Awareness of previously hidden strengths might, in turn, help them develop new skills for coping together effectively with both relational and nonrelational challenges in the middle and later years of life.

REFERENCES

Acock, A. C., & Schumm, W. R. (1993). Analysis of covariance structures applied to family research and theory. In P. G. Boss, W. J. Doherty, R. LaRossa, W. R. Schumm, & S. K. Steinmetz (Eds.), *Sourcebook of family theory and methods* (pp. 451-468). New York: Plenum.

Allen, K. R., & Walker, A. J. (1992). A feminist analysis of interviews with elderly mothers and their daughters. In J. F. Gilgun, K. Daly, & G. Handel (Eds.), *Qualitative methods in family research* (pp. 198-214). Newbury Park, CA: Sage.

Barnett, R. C. (1988). On the relationship of adult daughters to their mothers. *Journal of Geriatric Psychiatry, 21,* 37-50.

Baruch, G., & Barnett, R. C. (1983). Adult daughters' relationships with their mothers. *Journal of Marriage and the Family, 45,* 601-606.

Boyd, C. J. (1989). Mothers and daughters: A discussion of theory and research. *Journal of Marriage and the Family, 51,* 291-301.

Bromberg, E. M. (1983). Mother-daughter relationships in later life: The effect of quality of relationship upon mutual aid. *Journal of Gerontological Social Work, 6,* 75-92.

Bromberg, E. M. (1987). Mothers and daughters in later life: Rediscovery and renegotiation–A group work approach. *Journal of Gerontological Social Work, 11*, 7-24.

Cohler, B. J. (1988). The adult daughter-mother relationship: Perspectives from life-course family study and psychoanalysis. *Journal of Geriatric Psychiatry, 21*, 51-72.

Fischer, L. R. (1981). Transitions in the mother-daughter relationship. *Journal of Marriage and the Family, 43*, 613-622.

Fischer, L. R. (1986). *Linked lives: Adult daughters and their mothers.* New York: Harper and Row.

Hendricks, J. (1993). Recognizing the relativity of gender in aging research. *Journal of Aging Studies, 7*, 111-116.

Henwood, K. L. (1993). Women and later life: The discursive construction of identities within family relationships. *Journal of Aging Studies, 7*, 303-319.

Henwood, K. L., & Coughlan, G. (1993). The construction of "closeness" in mother-daughter relationships across the lifespan. In N. Coupland & J. F. Nussbaum (Eds.), *Discourse and lifespan identity: Language and language behaviors* (Vol. 4, pp. 191-214). Newbury Park, CA: Sage.

Mancini, J. A., & Blieszner, R. (1993, November). Aging parents and adult children: Cohesion, companionship, and conflict. In J. W. Dwyer (Chair), *Perspectives on the aging family and intergenerational exchanges.* Symposium presented at the annual meeting of the National Council on Family Relations, Baltimore.

O'Connor, P. (1990). The adult mother/daughter relationship: A uniquely and universally close relationship? *Sociological Review, 38*, 293-323.

Reinharz, S. (1986). Friends or foes: Gerontological and feminist theory. *Women's Studies International Forum, 9*, 503-514.

Rosenblatt, P. C., & Fischer, L. R. (1993). Qualitative family rescarch. In P. G. Boss, W. J. Doherty, R. LaRossa, W. R. Schumm, & S. K. Steinmetz (Eds.), *Sourcebook of family theory and methods* (pp. 167-177). New York: Plenum.

Scharlach, A. E. (1987). Role strain in mother-daughter relationships in later life. *The Gerontologist, 27*, 627-631.

Taylor, S. J., & Bogdan, R. (1984). *Introduction to qualitative research methods: The search for meanings* (2nd ed.). New York: Wiley.

Thompson, L. (1992). Feminist methodology for family studies. *Journal of Marriage and the Family, 54*, 3-18.

Thompson, L., & Walker, A. J. (1984). Mothers and daughters: Aid patterns and attachment. *Journal of Marriage and the Family, 46*, 313-322.

Troll, L. E. (1987). Mother-daughter relationships through the life span. In S. Oskamp (Ed.), *Applied social psychology annual: Vol. 7. Family processes and problems: Social psychological aspects* (pp. 284-305). Newbury Park, CA: Sage.

Troll, L. E. (1988). New thoughts on old families. *The Gerontologist, 28*, 586-591.

U. S. Bureau of the Census. (1982). *General population characteristics, Virginia* (PC80-1-B 48). Washington, DC: U. S. Government Printing Office.

Walker, A. J., & Thompson, L. (1983). Intimacy and intergenerational aid and contact among mothers and daughters. *Journal of Marriage and the Family,* *45,* 841-849.

Walker, A. J., & Thompson, L. (1984). Feminism and family studies. *Journal of Family Issues, 5,* 545-570.

Walker, A. J., Thompson, L., & Morgan, C. S. (1987). Two generations of mothers and daughters: Role position and interdependence. *Psychology of Women Quarterly, 11,* 195-208.

Weitzman, L. (1984). Sex-role socialization: A focus on women. In J. Freeman (Ed.), *Women: A feminist perspective* (3rd ed., pp. 157-327). Palo Alto, CA: Mayfield.

The Saliency
of the Grandmother-Granddaughter
Relationship:
Predictors of Association

Vira R. Kivett, PhD

SUMMARY. This study examined the solidarity of the grandmother-granddaughter tie when older women migrate. The sample, taken from a larger study ($N = 308$), included 69 relocated women with one or more grandchildren who reported a granddaughter to be the grandchild of most contact. The revised theory of intergenerational solidarity served as the conceptual framework. The results showed the saliency of the grandmother-granddaughter relationship depended upon the dimension examined. Tests of the hypotheses showed associational solidarity was primarily a function of the opportunity structure proximity and, to a smaller extent, age of the grandchild. No significant relationship existed between norms of grand filial expectations and affect for granddaughters and association. Neither did the results support the impact of norms on affect and their subsequent influence on association. *[Article copies available from The Haworth Document Delivery Service: 1-800-342-9678. E-mail address: getinfo@haworth.com]*

Vira R. Kivett is Excellence Professor in the Department of Human Development and Family Studies, School of Human Environmental Sciences, The University of North Carolina at Greensboro, Greensboro, NC 27412-5001.

[Haworth co-indexing entry note]: "The Saliency of the Grandmother-Granddaughter Relationship: Predictors of Association." Kivett, Vira R. Co-published simultaneously in the *Journal of Women & Aging* (The Haworth Press, Inc.) Vol. 8, Nos. 3/4, 1996, pp. 25-39; and: *Relationships Between Women in Later Life* (ed: Karen A. Roberto) The Haworth Press, Inc., 1996, pp. 25-39; and: *Relationships Between Women in Later Life* (ed: Karen A. Roberto) Harrington Park Press, an imprint of The Haworth Press, Inc., 1996, pp. 25-39. [Single or multiple copies of this article are available from the Haworth Document Delivery Service: 1-800-342-9678, 9:00 a.m. - 5:00 p.m. (EST). E-mail address: getinfo@haworth.com]

The grandmother-grandchild relationship is a normative and enduring connection important to most women. Typically, women enter the grandmother role during their middle years and can expect to spend nearly one-half of their lives as grandmothers. The grandmother-granddaughter relationship, in its voluntary form, provides many benefits to the older woman. It often contributes to women's feelings of biological renewal, emotional self-fulfillment, and vicarious accomplishment (Kivnick, 1981; Thomas, 1990). The actualization of the grandparent's role, however, requires interaction between grandparent and grandchild, such as shared time and space (Barranti, 1985) or an ongoing alliance to guarantee a "functional" relationship (Langer, 1990). We know little about the impact of distance on the grandparent-grandchild relationship when older grandparents move. The increasing number of older adults moving in retirement may have important implications for the grandparent-grandchild relationship.

The grandmother-granddaughter relationship has special salience in the intergenerational network despite little empirical evidence of the gender linkage. The significance of the female-to-female link can be extrapolated from the differential socialization of the sexes (Clingempeel, Colyar, Brand, & Hetherington, 1992) and the vertical generational bonds between females in lineages (Rosenthal, 1987). Women usually facilitate contact and carry out exchanges between generations (Barranti, 1985; Hagestad, 1985). As a result, women are more involved in families extended across generations and tend to have greater exchanges in female-to-female intergenerational links than men. Intergenerational ties, for example, are stronger among daughters, granddaughters, and grandmothers than among corresponding male links (Creasey, 1993; Hagestad, 1985). The maternal grandmother-granddaughter connection is more salient than other gender-linked grandparent-grandchild ties, followed by the maternal-grandfather tie, the paternal-grandmother tie, and the paternal-grandfather relationship (Roberto & Stroes, 1992). Additionally, research has shown an important relationship in the grandmother-granddaughter tie between older rural grandmothers and granddaughters (Kivett, 1993).

EXPLANATIONS
OF THE GRANDMOTHER-GRANDDAUGHTER TIE

Intergenerational Solidarity

The revised theory of intergenerational solidarity provides a framework for the examination of the grandmother-granddaughter relationship

(Bengtson & Roberts, 1991). The original theory draws upon classical theories of social organization, the social psychology of group dynamics, and the developmental perspective in family theory. It suggests that opportunity structure, familial norms, and kin affect are primary to kin association. An integral part of the refined theory is the specification of an interaction between normative expectations and kin affect in the explanation of family outcomes. This interaction is predicated upon the Gemeinschaft/ Gesellschaft distinction. That is, although small group dynamics have few normative expectations for affective and behavioral orientations, family dynamics have more extensive sets of expectations for affective and behavioral direction (Bengtson & Roberts, 1991). These expectations interact with affect to explain behavior.

The revised theory of intergenerational solidarity posits that: (a) opportunity for family intergenerational association will enable (or constrain) frequencies and types of association, (b) higher norms of familial primacy and higher levels of affect will lead to greater likelihood of intergenerational association, and (c) intergenerational affect and association will vary as a positive function of intergenerational norms of familism (Bengtson & Roberts, 1991). Previously, researchers applied the theory of intergenerational solidarity primarily to older parent-adult child groups. A modification of the refined theory served as the conceptual framework for the present study.

Opportunity structures for association. Several factors serve as either facilitators or barriers to the grandparent-grandchild relationship. The health of the grandparent often relates to the saliency of the grandparent's role. Adults with better physical and mental health play a more active role in the lives of their grandchildren (Baranowski, 1982; Hodgson, 1992; Kivett, 1993; Troll, 1985). Findings on the relationship between the age of the grandchild and the grandparent-grandchild relationship are equivocal. Some studies show a decrease in the grandparent-grandchild relationship with increased age of the grandchild (Barranti, 1985; Clingempeel et al., 1992; Thompson & Walker, 1987). Other researchers report increases in the relationship with increases in the age of the grandchild (Baranowski, 1982; Cherlin & Furstenberg, 1985; Hodgson, 1992; Nahemow, 1985).

Researchers have documented the importance of proximity to kin association and exchange (Bengtson & Roberts, 1991; Kivett, 1985a, 1988; Powers & Kivett, 1992). Findings consistently show the negative effect of distance upon the frequency of association and assistance. Geographical distance from grandchildren also heightens the ambiguity in the grandparent's role and its symbolic rather than functional nature (Matthews, 1984). Other opportunity structures for grandparent-grandchild association include: grandparents' relationships with intervening genera-tions (Barranti, 1985; Wentowski, 1985), frequent telephone contacts (Creasey, 1993; Kivett, Dugan, & Moxley, 1994), single marital status of the grandmother (Troll, 1985), and marital instability of the middle gen-eration (Clingempeel et al., 1992).

Grand filial norms. Research generally has shown a relative lack of norms regulating the grandparent-grandchild relationship (Johnson, 1983, 1985). Limited information on norms of grand filial expectations shows that grandparents have moderate norms of expectations for social support and low expectations for instrumental support (Langer, 1990; Powers & Kivett, 1992). Norms vary according to ethnicity, socioeconomic status, and familial need. The grandparent's role, particularly that of grandmoth-er, is more salient in ethnic than nonethnic families (Kivett, 1985b; Lub-ben & Becerra, 1987; Markides & Mindel, 1987). More flexible family structure is found in Black families that often include "fictive" grandchil-dren than in White families (Minkler & Roe, 1993). Problems in the lives of the younger generation, such as divorce, substance abuse, and incar-ceration, frequently redefine the normative expectations of the grandmoth-er's role (Dressel & Barnhill, 1994; Jendrek, 1994; Minkler & Roe, 1993; Troll, 1983).

Important interrelationships exist between normative expectations and family outcomes. Bengtson and Roberts (1991), in their refinement of the theory of intergenerational solidarity, argued the importance of norms to affect and intergenerational association. They posit that parents and chil-dren with strong commitment to familial norms will exhibit greater affec-tion for one another and have more extensive association.

Affect. Limited research shows high levels of grandparent affect for grandchildren. Kivett and associates (1994) found high levels of expressed affect for grandchildren of most contact among older migrants. Hodgson (1992) reported an important relationship between closeness of grandpar-ents and grandchildren and proximity to the grandchild. Grandchildren living nearer to their grandparents reported being closer to grandparents than those living at a distance. Other research, similarly, has shown high levels of affect between older rural adults and grandchildren (Powers & Kivett, 1992).

PURPOSE OF THE RESEARCH

This study examined the dynamics of the grandmother-granddaughter relationship when grandmothers move in retirement. Two primary ques-tions guided this research: (a) "What is the saliency of the grandmother-granddaughter relationship?", and (b) "What factors predict grandmother-granddaughter association?" The first hypothesis stated that proximity to granddaughters, good health of grandmothers, and younger granddaughters would predict high granddaughter association. The second hypothesis stated that high norms of grand filial expectations would predict high grandmother-granddaughter association. The third hypothesis posited that high affect for granddaughters would predict high association. The final hypothesis stated that high norms of grand filial expectations in combination with high affect would predict high association.

METHOD

Sample

The sample for this study was a subsample from a larger study of 308 adults 65 years of age or older who had moved either from another state or within the state since age 60. The subsample for the present study consisted of all the women in the study with one or more grandchildren who reported their grandchild of most contact to be a granddaughter ($N = 69$). In selecting the sample, a simple random procedure was used, incorporating compact cluster and random permutation techniques. In addition, "snowballing" techniques were used in several secured retirement communities. Group quarters were removed from the study population and sampled separately. The overall rejection rate was 32%.

Adults indigenous to the areas interviewed older adults in their homes. A 173-item questionnaire covered seven major areas: general information, migration motives, health, activities, family relationships, subjective well-being, and service use needs. Information was obtained on the family relations for the relative of most contact at six levels of kin. For purposes of the present study, I used only selected information on the granddaughter of most contact.

Measures

Dependent variable. The association scale consisted of seven items: doing things with the granddaughter (shopping, trips, movies), family gatherings for special occasions, eating together, visits, attending religious activities, writing, and telephoning. Possible responses ranged from daily (1) to never (10). Cronbach's standardized alpha for reliability was .87. Writing, originally included in the scale, was dropped because of its infrequency and negative effect upon the reliability coefficient.

Independent variables. Proximity to a grandchild was a functional measure with eight levels. Distances and coding ranged from living in the same household (1) to living 16 hours or more away (8). Health of grandmothers was a self-rated measure with a range of 0-9. Age of granddaughter was the actual age of the granddaughter at the time of the interview.

The scale measuring norms of grand filial expectations addressed five areas of assistance. Grandmothers reported on the extent to which they thought grandchildren should be responsible in providing services (shopping, driving, cleaning, and cooking), help in illness, financial assistance, visiting, and providing a home. Responses could range from never (1) to always (4). Cronbach's standardized alpha for reliability was .86.

Affect for the granddaughter was operationalized by obtaining a sum of the ratings respondents gave to their relationship with the granddaughter on five dimensions. Items included: getting along, communication, grandmother's understanding of the granddaughter, granddaughter's understanding of the grandmother, and feelings of closeness. Responses ranged from never (1) to always (6). Cronbach's standardized alpha of reliability was .90.

Statistical Procedures

Descriptive statistics (i.e., frequencies, percentages, and means) were used to analyze general information. Hierarchical multiple regression was used to test the hypotheses of the study. Association was regressed on the opportunity structures of proximity, health of grandmother, and age of granddaughter; norms of grand filial expectation; affect for the granddaughter, and a norms by affect interaction term.

RESULTS

Descriptive Findings

Of the 143 older women in the overall study having a grandchild, the majority, 54%, reported their grandchild of most contact was a granddaughter. The 69 grandmothers reporting a granddaughter of most contact had a mean of 5.26 grandchildren. Approximately 57% of granddaughters were daughters of grandmothers' child of most contact. Most grandmothers, 67%, had migrated for amenity reasons, usually climate. Approximately 57% of the women said their last move had not taken them away from family.

The average age of grandmothers was approximately 75 years (Table 1). They reported moderately high levels of health, education, and income. Most older women were married, 65%, with the unmarried being primarily widowed (96%). Approximately 9% had experienced multiple marriages. Most grandmothers (52%) lived within six hours of their grand-daughter of contact. The mean age of granddaughters was approximately 18 years (Table 1).

When the interviewers asked the grandmothers what they saw as their main role as a grandparent, they most frequently mentioned providing love and affection to grandchildren (45%); being there for the grandchild (30%) and providing help and advice (30%). Grandmothers had diverse

TABLE 1. Primary Characteristics of Migrated Grandmothers and Their Granddaughters of Most Contact

Characterstics	n	%	M
Marital status			
Married	45	65.2	
Unmarried	24	34.8	
Proximity			
Less than 30 minutes	11	15.9	
Less than 59 minutes	1	1.4	
1-3 hours	15	21.7	
4-6 hours	9	13.0	
7-10 hours	16	23.2	
11-15 hours	11	15.9	
16 plus hours	6	8.7	
Grandmother attributes			
Age			75.26
Education			14.01
Health			7.03
Income			$35–39,999
Granddaughter attribute			
Age			17.96
Others			
Grand filial expectations[a]			13.57
Granddaughter association[b]			38.21
Affect for granddaughter[c]			26.82

N = 69
[a]Range = 5–25
[b]Range = 6–60; higher scores = less association
[c]Range = 5–30

perceptions of their role, although they were usually of a noninstrumental nature. Responses ranged from demonstrations of affection and attention to baby-sitting. Grandmothers reported high affect for granddaughters (Table 1). They endorsed moderate norms of grand filial expectations. On a 10-point scale, grandmothers rated their satisfaction with their family relationships as 8.03 (not shown in table).

Grandmothers' association with granddaughters by traditional interpretations was moderately low as measured by face-to-face contact and telephoning (Table 1). As seen in Table 2, association was highest in visits followed by family gatherings and eating together. Grandmothers and granddaughters were less likely to attend religious activities together and to write to one another than other forms of association.

Tests of the Hypotheses

The results of the hierarchical multiple regression showed the model explained 51% of the variance in grandmother-granddaughter association ($R^2 = .51$, $F(6, 58) = 12.08$, $p < .001$) (Table 3). The first hypothesis, that the opportunity structures of proximity to granddaughters, good health of grandmothers, and younger granddaughters would predict high grandmother-granddaughter association, was partially supported. While proximity to granddaughters and granddaughters' age predicted higher association ($\beta = .46$, $p < .001$ and $\beta = .18$, $p < .05$, respectively), health of grandmothers was not related to frequency of association. A preliminary regression equation incorporating a quadratic term for age of granddaughter showed no curvilinear relationship between age and association (not shown).

The second hypothesis, that high norms of grand filial expectations would predict high grandmother-granddaughter association, was not supported. Similarly, the third hypothesis, that high affect for granddaughters would predict high association, was not supported. The fourth hypothesis also was not supported; high norms of grand filial expectations did not combine with high affect to predict high association.

CONCLUSIONS AND IMPLICATIONS

The grandmother-granddaughter relationship may serve both to anchor older women to changing social structures and to meet developmentally based imperatives. The maintenance of strong intergenerational bonds is of increasing concern given the growing numbers of older women who

TABLE 2. Types and Frequency of Association Between Migrated Grandmothers and Granddaughters of Most Contact

Frequency	Do things together	Family gatherings	Eat together	Visits	Religious activities	Writing letters[1]	Telephoning
			Types of Association				
Daily	0.0	0.0	0.0	2.9	1.4	0.0	2.9
Several times a week	4.3	2.9	2.9	5.8	1.4	0.0	11.6
About once a week	2.9	0.0	2.9	4.3	4.4	1.4	20.3
Several times a month	4.4	2.9	8.7	8.7	0.0	2.9	8.7
Once a month	1.4	1.5	5.8	2.9	1.4	13.0	11.6
Several times a year	44.9	59.4	53.6	49.4	20.4	26.2	23.3
About once a year	11.7	18.8	11.6	11.6	10.2	5.8	1.4
Every couple of years	2.9	4.4	4.4	4.3	2.9	0.0	0.0
Once a decade	0.0	0.0	0.0	0.0	1.5	0.0	0.0
Never	24.7	7.3	7.3	5.8	53.6	46.4	17.4
Missing	2.8	2.8	2.8	4.3	2.8	4.3	2.8

N = 69
[1]Dropped from the final scale because of low reliability.

TABLE 3. Regression of Grandmother-Granddaughter Association Upon Opportunity Structures for Interaction, Norms of Grand Filial Expectation, and Affect for Granddaughters

Step	Factor	R^2 (Adjustment)	R^2 Change	Sig. of Change	β
1	Opportunity structure				
	Grandmother's health				.05
	Grandmother's age				.18*
	Proximity	.23	.27	.000	.46***
2	Norms of grand filial expectations	.48	.25	.000	-1.09
3	Affect	.51	.04	.034	$-.46$
4	Norms x affect	.51	.01	.397	.68
	R^2 (adjusted) = .51, F (6,58) = 12.08***				

$^*p < .05;$ $^{***}p < .001$

migrate in retirement. The results of this study show that while most women migrants do not move away from family, most relocated grandmothers live seven or more hours away from their granddaughters of most contact. The saliency of the grandmother-granddaughter relationship has important implications for practitioners in strengthening the vital social connections of older women, particularly those individuals aging "out of place." The results of this study have several implications for strengthening the grandmother-granddaughter tie.

Increasing the Saliency of the Grandmother-Granddaughter Relationship

The importance of the grandmother-granddaughter relationship in migration depends upon the dimension of the relationship. The structural dimension of the relationship is high as it relates to the available pool of grandchildren and the frequency of granddaughters as the grandchild of most contact. This latter observation supports earlier findings of the primacy of vertical generational bonds between females in lineages (Clingempeel et al., 1992; Creasey, 1993; Hagestad, 1985).

The functional dimension of the grandmother-granddaughter relationship is moderately high as interpreted in the context of proximity to grandchildren. The finding that most relocated grandmothers associated with granddaughters several times a year, for example, may represent frequent interaction given the barrier of distance. The functional dimension of the relationship is moderately low, as reflected by grandmothers' broad range of perceived roles. Grandmothers, in general, viewed their most important roles as latent, nondescript relationships with granddaughters rather than active, instrumental roles. Although researchers have addressed the "normless" nature of the grandmother role (Johnson, 1983), norms of grand filial expectation may become more nondescript under constraints of geographical distance (Matthews, 1984).

The affectual dimension of the grandmother-granddaughter relationship is very high as seen through grandmothers' expressions of warmth and affection for granddaughters. Bengtson and Kuypers (1971) attribute high levels of affection expressed toward grandchildren to the "development stake" each generation holds for the younger generation. That is, the imperative of the older generation to transmit family values and legacies to successive generations. Central to this process are strong and enduring intergenerational bonds. Female-to-female transmissions may be a special imperative of older women (Rosenthal, 1987).

Practitioners should take both reactive and proactive positions in working with grandmothers whose roles have become obscured by distance or eliminated or weakened through divorce or other family dysfunction (Meyers & Perrin, 1993). A noteworthy number of grandmothers in the present study had divorce histories. Programs in adapting and transitioning to divorced and blended families, in maintaining family communication across distance, and "appropriate" and timely intrusion into the lives of grandchildren of divorce would be useful to older women. Educators and counselors can help strengthen weak grandmother-granddaughter relationships by assisting in the clarification of grandmother roles "at a distance." Also, grandmothers can be encouraged to develop more direct, nonmediated relationships with granddaughters. Similarly, they can enhance their relationships through increasing the amount of contact and one-on-one visits with granddaughters.

Enhancing Factors That Promote Grandmother-Granddaughter Solidarity

The results from this study suggest that theoretical models predicting older parent-child associational solidarity may vary according to intergenerational kin type and geographical mobility of the older adult. The findings do not support all tested posits of the revised theory of intergenerational solidarity. The data showed that grandmother-granddaughter solidarity in the case of migration is overwhelmingly a function of the opportunity structure, proximity. Other opportunity structures such as age of grand-daughter and health of grandmother are of little importance. Similarly, the data did not support the theoretical view of the important combined effect of norms of familism and affect for kin on association (the Gemeinschaft concept). Grandmothers with strong commitments to grand filial norms and high affect for granddaughters did not have more association with them than other grandmothers. This observation may relate to weak, non-descript norms of grand filial expectations or to the fact that proximity, as entered into the regression equation, controlled the relationships between norms and association and affect and association. In other words, norms of expectation and affect for granddaughters are of little consequence in grandmother-granddaughter association when opportunity structures such as proximity are considered.

These findings suggest that efforts to enhance grandmother-grand-daughter solidarity as viewed through association will be most useful by addressing the opportunity structure of proximity rather than affect and norms of expectation. Although researchers consistently report proximity as a major opportunity factor in kin outcomes, it explains considerably more variance when it is a major opportunity structure in the relationship such as in kin migration (Bengtson & Roberts, 1991; Kivett, 1985a, 1988; Powers & Kivett, 1992). Expanded use of telecommunications, as increasingly afforded through telephones, facsimiles, electronic mail, and video-phones, can enhance ties. Many older migrants are on the cutting edge of such technologies and frequently have the resources, orientation, and willingness to use more contemporary forms of communication.

Age of granddaughter also creates a small window of opportunity for association. This observation adds support to others' observations of the negative influence of age of grandchild on the grandparent-grandchild relationship (Barranti, 1985; Thompson & Walker, 1987). The finding of the unimportance of grandmothers' health to grandchildren association possibly relates to the lack of variability in older women's health ratings. Counselors and others might help older women in understanding development across the life span and, in particular, how they might better relate to the developmental needs and interests of granddaughters of various ages.

RESEARCH NEEDS

The results of this study suggest three major voids in the literature as it relates to grandmother-granddaughter relationships among newer cohorts of aging women such as older migrants. The first imperative is the need to develop theoretical models that explain intergenerational outcomes other than parent-child or traditional aging-in-place groups. These theories should address the increasing diversity of the population as it relates to ethnicity and social class. Theories may be generated best through ethnographic methodologies that capture the context of the relationship.

The second research imperative is the need to revisit older conceptual frameworks for their appropriateness in examining more contemporary grandmother-granddaughter relationships. Included here are dynamics between step-grandmothers and step-grandchildren, great-grandmothers and great-granddaughters, and adoptive and "fictive" granddaughters.

Finally, the third research imperative is the need to examine instruments traditionally used to measure familial norms, association, exchanges, and affect. Newly emerging normative regulations as a result of family dysfunction, social crises, and life style choices require that we revisit the norms associated with the grandparent-grandchild relationship. Emerging norms appear to be situation specific, strongly associated with ethnicity, "state-of" family, and the developmental interests and needs of grandparents.

REFERENCES

Baranowski, M. D. (1982). Grandparent-adolescent relations: Beyond the nuclear family. *Adolescence, 17,* 575-584.

Barranti, C. C. R. (1985). The grandparent/grandchild relationship: Family resource in an era of voluntary bonds. *Family Relationships, 34,* 343-352.

Bengtson, V. L., & Kuypers, J. A. (1971). Generational differences and the developmental stake. *Aging and Human Development, 2,* 249-260.

Bengtson, V. L., & Roberts, R. E. L. (1991). Intergenerational solidarity in aging families: An example of formal theory construction. *Journal of Marriage and the Family, 54,* 856-870.

Cherlin, A., & Furstenberg, F., Jr. (1985). Styles and strategies of grandparenting. In V. L. Bengtson & J. F. Robertson (Eds.), *Grandparenthood* (pp. 47-116). Beverly Hills, CA: Sage.

Clingempeel, W. G., Colyar, J. J., Brand, E., & Hetherington, E. M. (1992). Children's relationships with maternal grandparents: A longitudinal study of family structure and pubertal status effects. *Child Development, 63,* 1404-1422.

Creasey, G. L. (1993). The association between divorce and late adolescent children's relationships with grandparents. *Journal of Youth and Adolescence, 22,* 513-529.

Dressel, P. L., & Barnhill, S. K. (1994). Reframing gerontological thought and practice: The case of grandmothers with daughters in prison. *The Gerontologist, 34,* 685-691.

Hagestad, G. O. (1985). Continuity and connectedness. In V. L. Bengtson & J. F. Robertson (Eds.), *Grandparenthood* (pp. 173-181). Beverly Hills, CA: Sage.

Hodgson, L. G. (1992). Adult grandchildren and their grandparents: The enduring bond. *International Journal of Aging and Human Development, 34,* 209-225.

Jendrek, M. P. (1994). Grandparents who parent their grandchildren: Circumstances and decisions. *The Gerontologist, 34,* 206-216.

Johnson, C. L. (1983). A cultural analysis of the grandmother. *Research on Aging, 5,* 547-568.

Johnson, C. L. (1985). Grandparenting options in divorcing families: An anthropological approach. In V. L. Bengtson & J. F. Robertson (Eds.), *Grandparenthood* (pp. 81-96). Beverly Hills, CA: Sage.

Kivett, V. R. (1985a). Consanguinity and kin level: Their relative importance to the helping network of older adults. *Journal of Gerontology, 40,* 228-234.

Kivett, V. R. (1985b). Grandfathers and grandchildren: Patterns of association, helping, and psychological closeness. *Family Relations, 34,* 565-571.

Kivett, V. R. (1988). Older rural fathers and sons: Patterns of association and helping. *Family Relations, 37,* 62-67.

Kivett, V. R. (1993). Racial comparisons of the grandmother role: Implications for strengthening the family supports of older Black women. *Family Relations, 42,* 165-172.

Kivett, V. R., Dugan, E., & Moxley, S. C. (1994). *Family supports and relationships of older urban and rural migrants in North Carolina. Final Report to the AARP Andrus Foundation.* Greensboro, NC: The University of North Carolina at Greensboro.

Kivnick, H. Q. (1981). Grandparenthood and the mental health of grandparents. *Aging and Society, 1,* 365-391.

Langer, N. (1990). Grandparents and adult children: What do they do for one another? *International Journal of Aging and Human Development, 31,* 101-110.

Lubben, J. E., & Becerra, R. M. (1987). Social support among Black, Mexican, and Chinese elderly. In D. E. Gelfand & C. M. Barresi (Eds.), *Ethnic dimensions of aging* (pp. 130-142). New York: Springer Publishing Company.

Markides, K. S., & Mindel, C. H. (1987). *Aging and ethnicity.* Newbury Park, CA: Sage.

Matthews, S. H. (1984). The impact of divorce on grandparenthood: An exploratory study. *The Gerontologist, 24,* 41-47.

Minkler, M., & Roe, K. M. (1993). *Grandmothers as caregivers: Raising children of the crack cocaine epidemic.* Newbury Park, CA: Sage.

Myers, J. E., & Perrin, N. (1993). Grandparents affected by parental divorce: A population at risk? *Journal of Counseling and Development, 72,* 62-66.

Nahemow, N. (1985). The changing nature of grandparenthood. *Medical Aspects of Human Sexuality, 19,* 175-190.

Powers, E. A., & Kivett, V. R. (1992). Kin expectations and support among rural older adults. *Rural Sociology, 57,* 194-215.

Roberto, K. A., & Stroes, J. (1992). Grandchildren and grandparents: Roles, influences, and relationships. *International Journal of Aging and Human Development, 34,* 227-239.

Rosenthal, C. J. (1987). Generational successions: The passing on of family headship. *Journal of Comparative Family Studies, 18,* 61-77.

Thomas, J. L. (1990). Grandparenthood and mental health: Implications for the practitioner. *The Journal of Applied Gerontology, 9,* 464-479.

Thompson, L., & Walker, A. J. (1987). Mothers as mediators of intimacy between grandmothers and their young adult grandchildren. *Family Relations, 36,* 72-77.

Troll, L. E. (1983). Grandparents: The family watchdogs. In T. Brubaker (Ed.), *Family relationships in later life* (pp. 63-74). Beverly Hills, CA: Sage.

Troll, L. E. (1985). The contingencies of grandparenting. In V. L. Bengtson & J. F. Robertson (Eds.), *Grandparenthood* (pp. 135-149). Beverly Hills, CA: Sage.

Wentowski, G. W. (1985). Older women's perceptions of great-grandmotherhood: A research note. *The Gerontologist, 25,* 593-596.

Sisters in Later Life:
Changes in Contact and Availability

Jean Pearson Scott, PhD

SUMMARY. The strongest of sibling bonds is the relationship between sisters. However, researchers know little about how these relationships change over time. This study presents a longitudinal examination of structural and contact features of older, rural women's (N = 82) sibling networks. Also, sibling network variables were correlated with measures of subjective well-being. Significant loss of siblings occurred over 12 years. After controlling for proximity, frequency of contact between siblings did not change. Although sisters predominated in sibling networks, proximate brothers were slightly more prevalent and had more frequent contact with the respondents. Associations between sibling variables and subjective well-being were not found. Siblings remain active in the kin networks of women into late old age. *[Article copies available from The Haworth Document Delivery Service: 1-800-342-9678. E-mail address: getinfo@haworth.com]*

Popular songs, poems, and the visual media portray the close and intimate bond of sisters. A consistent body of empirical research on siblings is beginning to confirm this characterization. Regardless of age, sisters have the strongest sibling relationships in comparison to other gender combinations (Cicirelli, 1982).

Jean Pearson Scott is Professor, Department of Human Development & Family Studies, Texas Tech University, Lubbock, TX 79409.

This study was supported by a grant from the American Association of Family and Consumer Sciences, Alexandria, VA.

[Haworth co-indexing entry note]: "Sisters in Later Life: Changes in Contact and Availability." Scott, Jean Pearson. Co-published simultaneously in the *Journal of Women & Aging* (The Haworth Press, Inc.) Vol. 8, Nos. 3/4, 1996, pp. 41-53; and: *Relationships Between Women in Later Life* (ed: Karen A. Roberto) The Haworth Press, Inc., 1996, pp. 41-53; and: *Relationships Between Women in Later Life* (ed: Karen A. Roberto) Harrington Park Press, an imprint of The Haworth Press, Inc., 1996, pp. 41-53. [Single or multiple copies of this article are available from the Haworth Document Delivery Service: 1-800-342-9678, 9:00 a.m. - 5:00 p.m. (EST). E-mail address: getinfo@haworth.com]

Sibling relationships in later life are an increasingly important area of study because of the long duration of sibling ties over time, their shared family history, common memories that provide a basis for reminiscence, and their supportive role to each other. Siblings often must make decisions together and/or provide care to older parents in the final stages of life. Because of demographic changes, researchers anticipate that aged baby boomers will have more living siblings than adult children. This structural change will create more opportunity and perhaps greater need for sibling support than in previous generations (Gold, 1989).

One reason to specifically consider female sibling relationships in later life is the greater longevity of women and hence, the potential psychosocial support that female siblings as age peers can provide one another. Our understanding of female sibling ties in late old age is limited as is the available information regarding change in sibling relationships in later life. The purpose of this study, therefore, was to examine features of female sibling relationships in late old age, an age period defined for purposes of this study as age 75 and over, and to examine change in women's sibling relationships over time. Specifically, I examined structural features (e.g., number, availability, contact) because these variables may change as older women move into late old age and change the context of sister-sister interaction.

LITERATURE REVIEW

Although important work investigating the quality of sister-sister relationships (Adams, 1968; Cicirelli, 1982; Gold, 1989) and social support to sisters (Connidis, 1994; Matthews, Werkner, & Delaney, 1989; O'Bryant, 1988) exists, many studies of older siblings often do not include gender of both the respondent and the target sibling. Even fewer studies examine the gender composition of the sibling dyad or network or use the sibling dyad as the unit of analysis. The literature discussed in the following section pulls together previous work that specifically included an investigation of sisters or sister-sister dyads. I will examine gender both as an important individual characteristic and as a structural feature of a dyad or network.

There does not appear to be a relationship between sibling interaction in later life and general well-being for older adults, however, aspects of sister relationships have influenced well-being and psychological characteristics. Cicirelli (1980) found that older men with sisters had a greater sense of control in life and that women with sisters felt stimulated and challenged in their social roles. Structural features of sister relationships have positively influenced subjective well-being of older adults as well.

Structural Features of Sister Dyads

Connidis (1989) found several structural differences in her Canadian sample of older adults. Sisters were less likely than brothers to be married. Thus, sister pairs were more likely to have at least one single member or two previously married members. Marital status of dyad members was associated with other dyad characteristics. Dyads with at least one single member were closer geographically, were more likely to consider a sibling a close friend, and had more frequent face-to-face contact. In McGhee's (1985) study, having a proximate sister enhanced life satisfaction for older, rural women.

In addition to proximity, marital status of the sister and contact with her were important to both the support received and positive affect reported by recent widows (O'Bryant, 1988). Having a married sister nearby and having contact with her were significant predictors of positive affect. Having contact with an unmarried sister was most predictive of recent widows' support from their siblings.

Interaction Patterns of Sisters

There is limited evidence suggesting that a greater proportion of sister-sister dyads live closer together than other sibling combinations (Connidis, 1989). Also, sisters have greater face-to-face contact in comparison to other dyads (Connidis, 1989). Shanas (1973) observed that, with one exception (Yugoslavia), older women had greater face-to-face contact with siblings than older men in Western industrialized nations, Eastern Europe, and Israel. She attributed this gender difference to marital status, which predisposed more older women to being widowed and in need of support from extended kin.

Contact and Availability of Sisters in Rural Contexts

Of the limited studies comparing rural and urban samples on family interaction patterns, few differences emerge (Krout, 1986). The evidence regarding sibling relationships in rural contexts is sparse and virtually nil with respect to elderly sister ties.

Demographic data reveal differences in the composition of rural and urban elderly populations that relate to the availability of sisters in rural areas. Although women outnumber men in all old age groups (67 men for every 100 women 65+), the number of men is higher in rural areas (82.6 older men for every 100 older women) (Krout, 1986). This greater sex ratio in rural areas reflects occupational, marital status, and living arrangement patterns. The tendency for older, single women to move off farms accounts for the lower percentage of older widowed women in farm areas (28.5%) compared to those in nonfarm areas (51.8%) (Krout, 1986). Regardless of rural/urban designation, elderly women are more likely widowed and living alone than are elderly men. As expected, most elderly persons are married and male in rural versus urban settings. Thus, there is a lower probability of having a proximate female sibling in rural contexts. Data suggest that the mere availability of a sister may have positive implications for life satisfaction. When a sister was available, McGhee's (1985) older, rural women reported significantly higher life satisfaction than those who were without a proximate sister.

Older, rural respondents living in a North Carolina county reported an average of three living siblings with 86% having at least one sibling living within 49 miles of their home. Approximately 6% of the sample lived with a sister or brother (Kivett & Scott, 1979). In a thirteen-year follow-up of this sample, family visiting patterns were generally stable with most of the respondents having a weekly visit from siblings. Daily visiting increased over the 13-year interval. Only one in five persons had not seen a sibling within the year (Kivett & McCulloch, 1989).

In summary, gender and other structural features including (a) marital status of dyad members, (b) number and proximity of siblings, and (c) availability of other kin such as adult children, constrain or enable the sibling relationship. Due to the variations of methodologies and samples, researchers report inconsistencies in the influence of these structural characteristics on sibling interactions. Furthermore, few studies investigated sibling network characteristics across time or in rural contexts.

The present study sought to examine the structural features of the sibling network that form the context for supportive interactions. Based upon existing literature, I hypothesized that:

H_1 Sister-sister networks have greater face-to-face contact than other gender combinations.

H_2 Older, rural women with a proximate sister have greater levels of subjective well-being than women with distant sisters or near and distant brothers.

H_3 Over time, the size, proximity, and face-to-face contact of sisters with siblings of either gender decline.

METHOD

Sample

The sample included female participants (N = 82) from a larger study who participated in face-to-face interviews in 1981 and in 1993. Participants in the 1981 study were 65 years of age or older. The 1981 sample (N = 571) was randomly selected from a rural, two-county area in the Southwest through use of a compact cluster sampling technique. Approximately 24% of the original sample completed interviews at Time 2 (N = 135); of the remaining 75%, 53% had died, 20% had moved, and 3% refused to participate.

Trained interviewers contacted and interviewed participants in their own homes. A surrogate respondent completed the interview if the respondent was unable to answer questions; however, questions requiring subjective ratings were left unanswered. The majority of the rural women at Time 2 were Anglo (96.2%). They ranged in age from 76 to 96 years (M = 82.6). Their mean educational level was 10.2 years. Most of the women were widowed (82%) and lived alone (66%).

Measurement

The structural characteristics of the sibling network examined included: (a) number of living siblings, (b) number of living sisters, (c) number of living brothers, (d) proximity of brothers, (e) proximity of sisters, (f) frequency of contact with brothers, (g) frequency of contact with sisters, and (h) gender composition of the network. To measure *proximity of brothers and sisters,* respondents reported if they had a brother/sister living in the household, in the town or neighborhood, within 49 miles, within 50 to 250 miles, and over 250 miles. Numbers of brothers and sisters living at these distances were recorded at Time 2, and numbers of siblings undifferentiated by gender were recorded at Time 1. Similarly, the *frequency of contact* at Time 1 measurement was for sisters and brothers combined and the Time 2 measurement differentiated by gender. Respondents indicated how often the respondent had face-to-face contact with siblings who lived at each of four distances (for siblings living in the same household, daily contact was assumed). Possible responses for frequency of contact were: daily, weekly, monthly, several times a year, yearly, and less frequently. When several siblings lived the same proximity from the respondent, the interviewer recorded the one with the highest contact level. Similarly, at Time 2, if several sisters or brothers lived the same distance from the respondent, the interviewer recorded the highest level of contact. *Gender composition of the network* was sisters only, sisters with mixed gender siblings, and sisters with brothers only.

The *Philadelphia Geriatric Center Morale Scale* (PGCMS) (Lawton, 1975) and the *Center for Epidemiological Studies Depression Scale* (CES-D) (Radloff, 1977) were used to assess the subjective well-being of the respondents. The *PGCMS* is a 17-item multidimensional scale developed specifically for older respondents. The scale includes three factors: Agitation, Attitude Toward Own Aging, and Lonely Dissatisfaction. Morris and Sherwood (1975) found the scale to be reliably and structurally invariant across several dimensions in other samples of elderly persons. High scores reflect high morale. For the present sample, Cronbach's alpha was .82. A few studies present evidence for sensitivity to change in morale scores (George & Bearon, 1980). The mean morale scores in the present study were 12.3 and 12.5 at Times 1 and 2 respectively (scale ranged from 0 to 17).

The *CES-D* is a 20-item self-report scale designed to measure depressive symptomatology in the general population. Radloff (1977) reported internal consistencies (Cronbach alphas) of .85 to .90 and good criterion and construct-related validity. Respondents reported how often during the past week they felt symptoms of depressed mood (0) rarely (less than a day), to (3) most of the time (5-7) days. Researchers recommend the use of a total summed score; individuals with scores higher than 16 are "at risk" for clinical depression (Radloff, 1977; Thomas, Kelman, Kennedy, Ahn, & Yang, 1992). Cronbach's alpha for the present study was .79. The mean score at Time 2 was 7.7. Depression was not measured at Time 1.

RESULTS

Sister-Sister Ties

At age 75 and over, over two-thirds (65.9%) of the women in the present sample had one or more living sisters. Nearly a fifth (18.3%) of the women reported three or more living sisters (numbers ranging from 0 to 5). Despite having sisters, few sisters lived in the immediate vicinity (12.1%) (Table 1). Proximity to sisters clearly influenced frequency of face-to-face contact, however, the size of the sister network (one sister vs. two or more sisters) did not affect contact patterns (t-tests were nonsignificant). For sisters residing in the same town or neighborhood, visits were nearly weekly on average, nearly monthly for sisters living within 49

TABLE 1. Sibling Network Characteristics of Rural Older Women by Gender: Time 2

Variable		Brothers	Sisters
Number Living (%) (n=82)			
None		54.9	34.1
One		29.3	28.0
Two		9.8	19.5
Three or more		6.1	18.3
Number Living (M) (n= 60)		1.0	1.8***
At Least One Sib by Proximity (%) (n = 82)			
Household		0.0	1.2
Town/Neighborhood		13.4	10.9
Within 49 miles		4.9	10.9*
Within 50-250 miles		14.6	25.6**
Over 250 miles		28.0	32.9*
Frequency of Contact by Proximity (M) (n = 60)			
Town/Neighborhood		5.5	4.6
Within 49 miles		4.0	3.7
Within 50-250 miles		2.0	2.5
Over 250 miles		1.7	1.7
Network Composition (%) (N= 82)			
No Siblings	26.8		
Sister with Brothers	7.3		
Sister with Sisters and Brothers	37.8		
Sisters Only	28.0		

*$p < .05$; ** $p < .01$; ***$p < .001$

miles, once to several times a year for sisters living 50-250 miles from each other, and nearly yearly for those living over 250 miles away (Table 1).

Sibling Network Characteristics by Gender of Sibling

All data comparing sister-sister and sister-brother networks came from the Time 2 interviews. An initial observation is that these older women reported more living sisters (M = 1.8) than brothers (1.0) (t = 4.07, $p <$ .001). Considerably more women had three or more sisters (18.3%) in comparison to the percentage with three or more brothers (6.1%).

In comparing proportions of respondents with brothers and sisters by proximity, slightly more women reported a brother in comparison to a sister living in close proximity (in same town or neighborhood), however the difference was not significant. More older women reported having at least one sister living within 49 miles, within 50-250 miles, and over 250 miles in comparison to brothers (Table 1).

When controlling for proximity, sisters had more interaction with brothers in comparison to sisters for those whose sibling lived within 49 miles or closer, but the difference was not significant (Table 1). Unfortunately, cell sizes prevented more than tentative observations. Additional examination of the gender of the sibling network (sisters only, sisters with both sisters and brothers, and sisters with brothers only) indicated no differences in frequency of face-to-face contact. Thus, the data does not provide support for Hypothesis 1 (i.e., sisters would have greater face-to-face contact with sisters than with brothers) (Table 1).

Sibling Network Characteristics and Subjective Well-Being

To ascertain the possibility of associations between availability of siblings and subjective well-being, zero-order correlations were used to examine the relationship between: (a) number of sisters, (b) number of brothers, (c) proximity of sisters, (d) proximity of brothers, (e) frequency of contact with sisters, (f) frequency of contact with brothers, (g) morale, and (h) depression. Also, analysis of variance was used to examine the effect of gender composition of the sibling network on subjective well-being of older women. All correlations were small and nonsignificant. Furthermore, when comparing respondents with proximate sisters with those with proximate brothers, morale and depression scores did not differ. Thus, the data does not provide support for Hypothesis 2 (i.e., having a proximate sister would positively influence subjective well-being).

Network Characteristics over Time

At Time 1, 86% of older women in the present study reported having at least one living sister or brother (numbers ranging from 1 to 10) with an average of 3.5 siblings. Twelve years later, 72% of the women had at least one sibling (the range was from 1 to 7), with a mean of 2.3 living siblings. Although nearly three-fourths of the women had a sibling at Time 2, the number of siblings had declined significantly from Time 1 to Time 2 (Table 2).

With regard to availability of siblings at Times 1 and 2, there were more similarities than differences. A greater proportion of women reported having distant siblings than proximate ones and this held true for both time periods. However, even in late old age, approximately 23% of respondents had a sibling in the town or neighborhood (Table 3). Compared with the other distances, there was a greater decline from Time 1 to Time 2 in the proportion reporting a sibling living over 250 miles (Table 2).

TABLE 2. T1 vs. T2 Comparisons for Network Characteristics of Older Rural Women

Variable	Siblings	
	T1	T2
Number Living	3.5	2.3***
Number Living by Proximity		
Household (0)	- -	- -
In Town/Neighborhood (12)	1.7	1.3
Within 49 Miles (5)	1.2	1.0
Within 50-250 Miles (24)	2.0	1.6
Over 250 Miles (31)	2.9	1.8***
Proximity to Closest (#)	2.7	1.8***
Frequency of Contact (#)	3.6	3.2*
Frequency of Contact by Proximity		
In Town/Neighborhood (20)	5.3	5.3
Within 49 Miles (6)	4.0	3.5
Within 50-250 Miles (23)	2.7	2.3
Over 250 Miles (32)	1.8	1.8

Note. Paired t-tests were used for all analyses.
*p < .05; ***p < .001

As expected, the pattern of face-to-face contact with siblings clearly related to proximity of siblings. Most of the respondents had daily or weekly contact with siblings who lived in the town or neighborhood and yearly or less frequent contact with siblings living over 250 miles distance (Table 3). In comparing change in frequency of contact from Time 1 to Time 2, there were slight declines in the percentage of women reporting contact in comparison to Time 1, however, mean differences for frequency of contact were not significant (Table 2). As shown in Table 2, total contact scores were significantly lower at Time 2, however when controlling for proximity, no significant differences were found. In summary, the findings partially support Hypothesis 3 in that sibling network size declined significantly and distance to the closest sibling was greater on average. However, there was no reduction in their frequency of contact, after controlling for proximity.

DISCUSSION AND CONCLUSIONS

The present study examined structural and contact characteristics of the sibling networks of older, rural women over a 12-year period. Overall,

TABLE 3. Sibling Network Characteristics of Rural Older Women: Time 1 and 2

Network Variable	T1	T2
Percentage with One or More Sibs:		
In the Same Household	0.0	1.2
In Town/Neighborhood	29.1	22.5
Within 49 Miles	17.7	16.9
Within 50-250 Miles	46.8	39.4
Over 250 Miles	51.9	49.3
Frequency of Contact with Sibs Living:		
In Town/Neighborhood		
Daily or Weekly	91.0	82.4
Monthly/Several Times a Year	9.1	11.8
Yearly or Less Frequently	0.0	5.9
Within 49 Miles		
Daily or Weekly	20.0	15.4
Monthly/Several Times a Year	80.0	76.9
Yearly or Less Frequently	0.0	7.7
Within 50-250 Miles		
Daily or Weekly	5.4	0.0
Monthly/Several Times a Year	59.4	60.0
Yearly or Less Frequently	35.1	40.0
Over 250 Miles		
Daily or Weekly	0.0	0.0
Monthly/Several Times a Year	16.7	20.0
Yearly or Less Frequently	83.4	80.0

$N = 82$

siblings were an active component of the kin networks of older women through both their presence and loss, proximity, and contact even into late old age. The predominance of sisters in the sibling network reflects the advantage of longevity for women by providing sisters with a greater window of opportunity for interaction in late old age.

Despite the loss of brothers and sisters over time, frequency of interaction had not diminished which suggests that other siblings may have filled voids left by deceased siblings, particularly those siblings who lived at the same distance. The general pattern that emerges is one of a "thinning" of the sibling networks of these older, rural sisters.

An unanticipated finding was the greater percentage of women who had a proximate brother (13.4%) in comparison to a sister (10.9%) and the correspondingly greater contact with proximate brothers (M = 5.5) in comparison to sisters (M = 4.6). This finding may reflect the rural setting of the study where ranching and farming, typically male-dominated occupations, predominate. In agricultural areas, males may have greater reason to remain in the area to operate the family ranch or farm (Krout, 1986). Women of late old age may rely on brothers who live nearby to maintain their independence in sparsely populated agricultural regions. However, I did not examine patterns of assistance among siblings in the present study. Nevertheless, the women's reports of daily to weekly face-to-face contact with their brothers suggested that they had the opportunity to exchange assistance and/or social-emotional support.

The lack of associations between sibling network variables and measures of subjective well-being supported the findings of Lee and Ihinger-Tallman (1980), but did not support more recent studies (McGhee, 1985; O'Bryant, 1988). For example, McGhee's rural study found presence and availability of sisters to be important to life satisfaction; this relationship was not found for the sisters in the present study. The generally high levels of morale and low depression scores of these older women may have limited the role that siblings might ordinarily have in boosting subjective well-being.

In conclusion, although the loss of network members affects sibling networks, patterns of contact between siblings remain stable. Availability influences face-to-face contact with siblings with no evidence of a preference for female siblings. Other than the preponderance of sisters in women's sibling networks, proximity and contact do not reveal the greater salience of sisters in comparison to brothers in women's sibling networks in late old age. Indeed, within the rural context of the present study, greater availability of proximate brothers was found.

IMPLICATIONS FOR FUTURE RESEARCH AND PRACTICE

The women in the present study were primarily Caucasian and lived in a sparsely populated rural region of the Southwest, thereby limiting the generalizability of the findings. How structural features of sibling networks either enable or constrain supportive ties among sisters particularly among old- and oldest-old women warrants further attention. In addition, the findings of the present study were limited to structural and contact data. We need more information regarding support and qualitative aspects of sisters' relationships in varying rural/urban contexts. Marital status of sisters, which was a differentiating feature of support in O'Bryant's (1988) study of older widows, is a variable warranting further investigation in a rural context.

Despite the loss of siblings in advanced old age, surviving sisters and sister-brother ties remain relatively stable in a remote rural location. Service providers and practitioners should ask elderly clients about sibling availability, contact, and nature of support and view these ties as potential resources to complement other family or formal support. Ensuring that older siblings have a telephone adapted for hearing or vision impairment or have transportation for visits could enhance sibling interaction. Efforts to maintain sibling contact may facilitate reminiscence and resolution of sibling losses. Interaction with surviving siblings to resolve sibling losses may be important to the overall emotional adjustment of persons in late old age and needs further investigation.

REFERENCES

Adams, B. N. (1968). *Kinship in an urban setting.* Chicago: Markham.

Cicirelli, V. G. (1980). Sibling relationships in adulthood: A life-span perspective. In L. W. Poon (Ed.), *Aging in the 1980s: Psychological issues* (pp. 455-462). Washington, DC: American Psychological Association.

Cicirelli, V. G. (1982). Sibling influence throughout the lifespan. In M. E. Lamb & B. Sutton-Smith (Eds.), *Sibling relationships: Their nature and significance across the life span* (pp. 267-284). Hillsdale, NJ: Erlbaum.

Connidis, I. A. (1989). Siblings as friends in later life. *American Behavioral Scientist, 33,* 81-93.

Connidis, I. A. (1994). Sibling support in older age. *Journals of Gerontology, 49,* S309-S317.

George, L., & Bearon, L. (1980). *Quality of life in older persons.* New York: Human Sciences.

Gold, D. T. (1989). Generational solidarity: Conceptual antecedents and consequences. *American Behavioral Scientist, 33,* 19-32.

Kivett, V. R., & McCulloch, B. J. (1989). *Support networks of the very-old: Caregivers and carereceivers (Caswell III).* Greensboro, NC: University of North Carolina, School of Human Environmental Sciences, Family Research Center.

Kivett, V. R., & Scott, J. P. (1979). *The rural by-passed elderly: Perspectives on status and needs* (Tech. Bulletin No. 260), North Carolina Agricultural Research Service, Raleigh; University of North Carolina, Greensboro.

Krout, J. A. (1986). *The aged in rural America.* New York: Greenwood.

Lawton, M. P. (1975). The Philadelphia Geriatric Center Morale Scale: A revision. *Journal of Gerontology, 30,* 85-89.

Lee, G. R., & Ihinger-Tallman, M. (1980). Sibling interaction and morale. *Research on Aging, 2,* 367-391.

Matthews, S. H., Werkner, J. E., & Delaney, P. J. (1989). Relative contributions of help by employed and unemployed sisters to their elderly parents. *Journal of Gerontology, 44,* S36-S44.

McGhee, J. L. (1985). The effects of siblings on the life satisfaction of the rural elderly. *Journal of Marriage and the Family, 47,* 85-91.

Morris, J. N., & Sherwood, S. (1975). A retesting and modification of the Philadelphia Geriatric Center Morale Scale. *Journal of Gerontology, 30,* 77-84.

O'Bryant, S. (1988). Sibling support and older widows' well-being. *Journal of Marriage and the Family, 50,* 173-183.

Radloff, L. (1977). The CES-D Scale: A self-report depression scale for research in the general population. *Applied Psychological Measurement, 1,* 385-401.

Shanas, E. (1973). Family-kin networks and aging in cross-cultural perspective. *Journal of Marriage and the Family, 35,* 505-511.

Thomas, C., Kelman, H., Kennedy, G., Ahn, C., & Yang, C. (1992). Depressive symptoms and mortality in elderly persons. *Journal of Gerontology, 47,* S80-S87.

Friendships Between Older Women: Interactions and Reactions

Karen A. Roberto, PhD

SUMMARY. The purpose of this study was to examine specific interactions between older women and multiple members of their close friend network. Ninety-four women, 65 years of age and older, described their interactions with 182 close friends. The women reported substantial social and emotional involvement with their close friends. Almost all of the women reported getting together with their close friends "just to talk." For women with multiple close friends, the topics of these conversations differed depending on which friends the women described. Perceptions of equity and inequity in their relationships influenced the way in which the women described their friends and the feelings they expressed about their friendships. *[Article copies available from The Haworth Document Delivery Service: 1-800-342-9678. E-mail address: getinfo@haworth.com]*

Friendships play a significant role in the personal and social lives of most women (cf. Blieszner & Adams, 1992; Fehr, 1996; O'Connor, 1992; Oliker, 1989). Throughout adulthood, women turn to their close friends for personal, emotional, and affective support. They share intimate information and participate in instrumental and social activities with their

---

Karen A. Roberto is Director, Center for Gerontology, Virginia Polytechnic Institute and State University, Blacksburg, VA 24061-0426.

The collection of data used for this study was funded by the Radcliffe Research Support Program, Henry A. Murray Research Center, Radcliffe College, Cambridge, MA while the author was a Visiting Scholar at the Center.

[Haworth co-indexing entry note]: "Friendships Between Older Women: Interactions and Reactions." Roberto, Karen A. Co-published simultaneously in the *Journal of Women & Aging* (The Haworth Press, Inc.) Vol. 8, Nos. 3/4, 1996, pp. 55-73; and: *Relationships Between Women in Later Life* (ed: Karen A. Roberto) The Haworth Press, Inc., 1996, pp. 55-73; and: *Relationships Between Women in Later Life* (ed: Karen A. Roberto) Harrington Park Press, an imprint of The Haworth Press, Inc., 1996, pp. 55-73. [Single or multiple copies of this article are available from the Haworth Document Delivery Service: 1-800-342-9678, 9:00 a.m. - 5:00 p.m. (EST). E-mail address: getinfo@haworth.com]

55

friends. For older women, friendships provide the opportunity for the exchange of intimacy, emotional support, and assistance.

Researchers report moderate to high levels of homogeneity within the friendship networks of older women (Babchuk & Anderson, 1989; Dykstra, 1990; Usui, 1984). Women typically name other women as their close friends. They are of approximately the same age and socioeconomic status, share the same racial/ethnic background, and live within the same geographic location. The quantity and quality of interactions between older women and their friends differ, however, depending upon the specific characteristics of the friendship. A summary of comparative data suggests that there are differences in later life friendships based on the construction of the definition of friendship (e.g., researchers vs. study participants), the level of the relationship under investigation (e.g., close friends vs. casual friends), and the focus of the analysis (e.g., friend dyad vs. global friendships) (Adams, 1989). Within these parameters, researchers typically gather information about interactions between friends by having respondents focus on a particular friend or group of friends; there is limited information available about the specific relationships between older women and their friends within the same friendship categories (e.g., best friends). The findings of a recent study suggest that, to a certain extent, the qualities older women use to characterize their close friend relationships depend upon the friendship being examined (Roberto, 1996). Even when using the same framework for defining friends, it appears that not all close friendships are alike; thus reinforcing the personal nature of the friend relationship.

In this paper, I examine specific interactions between older women and multiple members of their close friend network to further explore similarities and differences in close friend relationships. I begin with a brief overview of the literature describing the interaction patterns (i.e., instrumental, social, affective) of older adults and their friends. Then, using data from a survey of 94 older women, I present information on: (a) what older women and their close friends do for one another, (b) the type of social activities they engage in, (c) the topics of their conversations, and (d) the older women's reactions to their friendships. The paper ends with a discussion of the findings and implications for future practice and research.

INTERACTIONS BETWEEN FRIENDS IN LATER LIFE

Instrumental Support

Most older adults report that, if they need assistance, they have friends they can turn to for help. Yet, in the course of daily life, friends provide limited assistance to one another. When examining the instrumental support patterns of older women and their friends, transportation is the most frequent type of help exchanged (Adams, 1985/86; Armstrong & Goldsteen, 1990; Roberto & Scott, 1984/85; Scott & Roberto, 1987). Other common types of assistance include short-term services (e.g., running errands, minor household repairs) and help during times of brief illnesses.

The degree to which older friends provide support for each other depends on the constellation of their circumstances (Allan, 1989). Factors such as marital status, health, living arrangements, and the availability of family members and formal services influence the helping relationship between friends. For example, individuals not married in their later years report more frequent contact with their friends and rely more heavily on friends for instrumental support than do their married counterparts (Essex & Nam, 1987; Roberto & Scott, 1984/85). Healthy older adults appear to maintain a balance of giving and receiving instrumental support within their friendships whereas older individuals who perceive themselves in poorer health than their friends are more likely to be on the receiving end of the relationship (Goodman, 1985; Johnson & Troll, 1994; Roberto & Scott, 1986). Older women living in rural areas more actively engage in the exchange of assistance (e.g., assistance when ill, shopping) with members of their friend network than their urban counterparts (Scott & Roberto, 1987).

Social Activities

Friendships in later life provide the opportunity for companionship and sociability that older adults find rewarding (Allan, 1989; O'Connor, 1992). Attending and participating in activities of local organizations, clubs, churches, and senior recreation centers provide older women the opportunities for socializing with friends (Adams, 1987) and integrate older adults into the community (Nussbaum, Thompson, & Robinson, 1989). The types of activities older friends engage in is a function of their personal interests as well as the opportunities that are available to them. For example, a study of the friendship patterns of older adults living in urban and rural areas found that more urban women participated in drop-in visits, commercial activities, and happy occasions such as birthdays and holidays with friends, whereas rural women seemed more involved in home and outdoor recreational activities (Roberto & Scott, 1987). The authors suggested that lack of formal programs and events in rural areas, as well as the physical distance between individuals, may influence the type of social interactions between friends.

Affective Support

For most older women, friendships require time purely for direct dialogue or shared conversation. These conversations reinforce the intimate and expressive components of women's friendships. Past research provides limited information, however, about what older women talk about with their friends. Topics discussed by young-adult and middle-aged women and their close friends include personal problems, marital and family relationships, daily activities, community/civic affairs, personal network news and activities, and their emotions, need for autonomy and individuality (Johnson & Aries, 1983; Oliker, 1989). Older women also report sharing thoughts and feelings with their close friends. They tell them things that they do not share with anyone else (Dykstra, 1990; Lewittes, 1989). These conversations, however, typically focus on everyday things and family activities rather than individual concerns and feelings. For older women who recently lost their spouse, extensively talking about their experience with friends often strengthens the bond between them (Rawlins, 1992). This intensive focus on personal issues and concerns, however, tends to be short-term.

REACTIONS TO RELATIONSHIPS WITH CLOSE FRIENDS

Older women's interactions with their friends influence their perceptions of and satisfaction with their friendships. On a relationship level, equity, or the perceived balance of giving and receiving, is an important concept to consider when examining the reactions of older women to their friendships. According to the tenets of equity theory, individuals are most satisfied with their relationships when they perceive them as equitable (Walster, Walster, & Berscheid, 1978). When individuals participate in inequitable relationships they become distressed and report being less content and satisfied with their relationships. These negative feelings motivate the individual either to attempt to restore fairness in their relationship or, in extreme cases, terminate the relationship.

On a personal level, perceiving one's friendship as equitable or inequitable effects the feelings expressed by older women. Older persons involved in friendships in which they perceive themselves as receiving more from the relationship than giving to it (i.e., overbenefited) report feeling greater amounts of anger and distress than those who are giving more than they are receiving (i.e., underbenefited) or those in more reciprocal relationships (Roberto & Scott, 1986; Rook, 1987). Researchers have not determined, however, if perceiving one's friendship as equitable or inequitable differentiates older women's beliefs and feelings about their friends.

METHOD

Sample

The sample for this study stems from the *McBeath Institute–Aging Women Project, University of Wisconsin–Madison*. The original project examined issues affecting women as they aged (e.g., social and intimate relationships, life events, organizational and recreational activities, and physical and psychological health). In 1978, researchers interviewed a random, representative sample of 480 women drawn from the total Madison population of women 50 years of age and older.[1] During year two of the project (1979), 400 (83%) of the original women were re-interviewed.

In 1992, I conducted a follow-up study of a sub-sample (n = 110) of these women. The purpose of this study was to examine older women's friendships over time. The Henry A. Murray Research Center at Radcliffe College made available the coded data from the original interviews. I obtained the women's names, addresses, phone numbers, and names of their close friends from the files of original investigators and verified the information with Madison's telephone and city directories. The city and county death records were reviewed in an attempt to identify women not located.

Procedure

To reach the targeted sample size of 100 women with at least one close friend, I contacted approximately 30% of the original sample members using a two-step sampling procedure. All potential participants received a letter from the original investigators explaining the purpose of this study and the possibility that they may be re-contacted. Approximately one week after sending the letters, I began contacting the women by phone to request their participation in the study. Initial participation required the women to complete a phone interview, lasting approximately 20 minutes.

During the original study, the researchers asked the women to identify, by first name, their closest friend in 1978 and their two closest friends in

---

1. See Roberto (1996) for a detailed explanation of the original sampling procedure used to select the women.

1979. During the 1992 follow-up, I asked the women to name their closest friend. If the women did not name a friend previously identified, I asked them if that person was still a close friend. If, during the 1978-79 interviews, the women named multiple close friends I asked about the status of each friendship. At the end of the phone interview, I also asked the women if they had made any new close friends within the last 10-15 years. If they said yes, demographic information was gathered for this friendship (e.g., when they met; how they met; why they considered them a close friend).

Upon completion of the phone interview, I asked the women to complete a more in-depth questionnaire about themselves and their current interactions with their close friends. The women received a stipend of five dollars for completing the additional questionnaire. Ninety-five of the 102 women naming a close friend (eight women said that they currently did not have anyone with whom they were close friends) completed and returned a usable questionnaire for a response rate of 93%. The information received from 94 women naming only women as their close friends and completing both the phone survey and mailed questionnaire was analyzed for this paper. Overall, the women had the opportunity to discuss their relationships with five friends. Thirty-four percent (n = 32) of the women reported on one close friendship, 44.0% (n = 42) described two close friendships, 17.0% (n = 16) discussed three close friendships, and 5.0% (n = 5) of the women described their relationship with four close friends.

Measures

As part of the mailed questionnaire, the women completed a series of social network questions concerning the instrumental, social, and affective aspects of their friendships. These questions were drawn from literature on older adult friendships (cf. Adams & Blieszner, 1989; Blieszner & Adams, 1992). The women responded either (0) no or (1) yes to each question. The women reported on their exchange of *instrumental assistance* by indicating if, during the last six months, they provided help to or received help from their close friends in the following areas: transportation, shopping, running errands, finances, housekeeping, household, and loaning household items. The women also indicated if they participated in any of the following *social activities* with their close friends: getting together for conversation, going to movies/concerts, playing cards/board games, going out to dinner, dining at home, going to sports events, going on vacations, watching television, attending club/organization meetings, participating in senior center activities, participating in sports, taking walks/drives, going shopping, celebrating special occasions, and exchanging gifts. The women assessed the *affective* component of their friendship by indicating what they talked about (i.e., self-disclosure) with their friends. The women reported if they shared or discussed the following topics: family problems, health problems, financial concerns, problems with other friends, happy family events, sad family events, mundane details of everyday life, gossip, death and dying, sexuality, morals and values, religious beliefs, political views, opinions about current events, feelings of joy, feelings of anger, fears, personal feelings, and personal secrets.

Items also included in the questionnaire assessed the women's feelings and perceptions about their friendships and their friends. A modified version of the *Walster Global Measure of Participants' Perceptions of Inputs, Outcomes, and Equity/Inequity* (Walster, Walster, & Berscheid, 1978) measured the women's perception of equity within their friendships. The women rated their own and their friends' contributions to their relationship. For example, the women responded to the following question: "Taking all things into consideration (i.e., how much you help each other, the kinds of things you share with each other, etc.), how would you describe *your contributions* (what you give) to your friendship?" The women then described their own and their friend's outcomes from their friendship: "Taking all things into consideration (i.e., how much you help each other, the kinds of things you share with each other, etc.), how would you describe *your friend's outcomes* (what he/she gets) from your friendship?" Response categories for each of the four questions ranged from (1) extremely low to (8) extremely high.

Equity was calculated using the linear formula proposed by Harris (1983):

$$(O_A - aI_A) - (O_B - aI_B).$$

In this formula A and B refer to the outcomes and inputs, respectively, and *a* is a parameter taking on a value between 0 and 1 (chosen on a prior grounds). Harris (1983) states that setting *a* between these two extremes results in the most accurate index of equity; *a* was set at 0.5. Based on their equity scores, I coded the women's friendships as either *overbenefited* (the women's relative outcomes/inputs were higher than their friends), *equitable* (i.e., a balance of outcomes/inputs for both the older women and their friends) or *underbenefited* (i.e., the women's outcomes/inputs were lower than their friends).

To determine the influence of perceived equity on the women's friendships, the women completed a modified version of *Austin's Total Mood Index* (cited in Walster et al., 1978). The women responded to the following question(s): "When you think about how much you do for your friends and how much they do for you, to what extent do you feel content and happy (angry, guilty, grateful)?" Responses for each item were coded (1) not at all, (2) a little, (3) somewhat, and (4) very much. To explore if there were differences in how the women described or felt about their friends, based on their perceptions of equity within their friendships, they responded (0) no or (1) yes to the following three questions: "Would you describe your close friend as someone who (a) is comfortable to be around; (b) sometimes makes me feel bad or gets me down; and (c) is someone I consider as close as family?"

Analysis

Nonparametric statistics were used to compare the interactions of women who reported on their relationship with multiple friends.[2] The McNemar test detects significant differences in the proportion of women reporting on their relationship with two close friends. This test uses a binomial distribution to compute significance level if differences occur in fewer than 30 cases (Siegel & Castellan, 1988). Cochran Q analysis tests for significant differences in the proportion of women describing their interactions with three close friends. Separate analyses were not done for women with four close friends due to the small sample (n = 5 women).

A series of one-way analysis of variance was conducted to detect differences in how the older women felt about their friendships according to their perceptions of equity within the relationships. When calculating the ANOVA's, the harmonic mean of the sample was used because the n's were not equal in all three groups. Duncan Multiple Range tests were used to determine differences among the three groups of women when overall significance occurred. Chi-square analyses were used to examine differences in the women's feelings about their friends according to their perceptions of equity within the relationships. These analyses were performed for the overall sample of friendships. A statistical examination of the reactions of women with two and three close friends was not possible because of the small sample and the skewed distribution of equity scores.

---

2. For women with multiple close friends, the designation of friendship 1, 2, and 3 was assigned based on the order in which the women first discussed their friends with the researcher; the terms *do not* refer to any preference the women may have had for one close friend over the other. These same friendships are referred to throughout the rest of this manuscript whenever comparisons are made.

RESULTS

Characteristics of the Women and Their Close Friends

The women ranged in aged from 65 to 89 (M = 73.9; S.D. = 6.2). Forty-five percent of the women currently were married, 38.0% were widowed, 7.0% were divorced, and 10.0% never married. The women had a mean educational level of 13.8 years (S.D. = 3.2). Thirteen percent of the women currently worked outside the home, 58.0% regarded themselves retired, and 29.0% considered themselves homemakers. The gross annual income of the women ranged from between $5000 to $9999 (8.0%) to over $25,000 (36.0%). When asked about the status of their health, approximately 22.0% reported their health as excellent, 46.0% said it was good, 22.0% responded that they were in fair health, and 10.0% rated their overall health as poor. Forty-three percent of the women reported that their health did not prevent them from doing the things they wanted to, whereas 40.0% said that their health stood in their way of doing things a little or some of the time, and 17.0% responded that their health stood in the way of doing the things they wanted to a great deal of the time.

The women reported currently having an average of five (S.D. = 7.4) close friends. The close friends they discussed for the follow-up study ranged in age from 26 to 95 (M = 68.9; S.D. = 11.8). They knew these close friends an average of 29 years (S.D. = 19.9). Most women had frequent contact with their close friends. Fifty percent of the women and their close friends had face-to-face visits at least once a week and 58.0% talked on the phone at least once a week.

Interactions with Close Friends

Assistance. The women provided and received limited help from their close friends. They most frequently reported giving help to and receiving help from their friends in the areas of transportation, shopping, and running errands (Table 1). When comparing the responses of women who reported on their instrumental activities with two close friends (FR1 and FR2), no significant differences occurred for providing help. However, the women were more likely to receive help in the area of "running errands" from FR1 than from FR2 ($p < .05$). No other significant differences were found in the proportion of women receiving assistance from either friend. For women with three close friends (FR1, FR2, and FR3), a greater proportion of women provided transportation to FR1 than FR2 or FR3 ($Q = 10.67$, $p < .01$). No other significant differences were found in the proportion of women giving help to or receiving help from their three close friends.

TABLE 1. Percentage of Women Giving Help To and Receiving Help From Close Friends

Type of Help	All Friendships (n = 180)	Two Friends (n = 40)		Three Friends (n = 16)		
		FR1	FR2	FR1	FR2	FR3
GIVING HELP						
Transportation	36.9	42.5	32.5	62.5	12.5	37.5
Shopping	23.3	32.5	17.5	18.8	12.5	18.8
Running Errands	19.9	22.5	10.0	25.0	18.8	25.0
Loaning Items	15.6	10.0	17.5	18.8	0.0	6.3
Housekeeping	5.7	7.5	2.5	12.5	0.0	0.0
Finances	4.6	5.0	2.5	12.5	0.0	0.0
Household Repairs	4.0	5.0	5.0	6.3	6.3	6.3
RECEIVING HELP						
Transportation	40.2	45.5	38.5	43.8	37.5	31.3
Shopping	19.0	27.5	15.8	18.8	6.3	6.3
Running Errands	21.2	30.0	10.0	31.3	6.3	25.0
Loaning Items	10.6	10.0	7.5	18.8	0.0	6.3
Housekeeping	6.1	2.5	4.9	12.5	0.0	0.0
Finances	3.3	2.5	0.0	6.3	0.0	0.0
Household Repairs	3.3	5.0	7.5	0.0	0.0	6.3

Social Activities. The most common social activity that the women and their close friends participated in was getting together for conservation (Table 2). This occurred in 92.0% of the friendships. Going out to dinner was a common activity for almost three-fourths of the friends. In addition, celebrating special occasions, exchanging gifts, and dining at each other's homes were common occurrences in over 50% of the friendships. The least common activities shared by friends were going to the senior center (7.6%) and participating in sporting events (6.0%). Significant differences were found for three activities for women reporting on two close friendships. A greater proportion of women go to movies, plays or concerts (p < .05), go for walks or drives (p < .01), and go shopping (p < .05) with FR1 than FR2. One significant difference was found for women with three close friends. A greater proportion of women vacationed with FR1 and FR3 than with FR2 (Q = 8.00, p < .05). In addition, differences ap-

TABLE 2. Percentage of Women Participating in Activities with Close Friends

Activity	All Friends (n = 182)	Two Friends (n = 41)		Three Friends (n = 16)		
		FR1	FR2	FR1	FR2	FR3
Conversation	92.2	90.2	95.1	87.5	81.3	62.5
Go Out to Dinner	72.3	90.2	75.6	81.3	50.0	62.5
Celebrate Sp. Occasions	57.9	65.9	53.7	81.3	37.5	50.0
Exchange Gifts	55.2	65.9	56.1	81.3	56.3	43.8
Dine at Home	51.6	65.9	48.8	68.8	37.5	43.8
Walks/Drives	48.4	63.4	36.6	56.3	37.5	43.8
Movies/Concerts	43.5	61.0	31.7	62.5	31.3	43.8
Shopping	42.6	56.1	36.6	43.8	25.0	25.0
Club/Org. Mtgs.	35.9	41.5	39.0	43.8	25.0	50.0
Cards/Board Games	34.8	34.1	31.7	56.3	31.3	37.5
Watch TV	25.5	22.0	17.1	25.0	12.5	6.3
Vacations	23.4	36.6	22.0	37.5	0.0	25.0
Attend Sports Events	10.9	22.0	7.3	0.0	6.3	12.5
Senior Center	7.6	4.9	4.9	12.5	6.3	25.0
Part. in Sports	6.0	4.9	4.9	12.5	0.0	12.5

proached significance for four additional activities: playing cards/games ($Q = 5.09$), dining at each other's homes ($Q = 5.43$), celebrating special occasions ($Q = 5.25$), and exchanging gifts ($Q = 5.20$) (all p values = .07). For each activity, a greater proportion of women were more likely to participate with FR1 than with FR2 and FR3.

Self-Disclosure. As shown in Table 3, the most common topics shared between the women and their close friends were happy and sad events within their families, feelings of joy, and health problems. The most common things "never" shared within the friendships were the women's views on sexuality and their most personal secrets. When comparing the responses of women who reported on their relationships with two close friends, significant differences occurred for only three topics of discussion. A greater proportion of women discussed their views on sexuality ($p < .01$), their religious beliefs ($p < .05$), and their fears ($p < .05$) with FR1 than with FR2. For women with three close friendships, significant differences occurred for 10 of the 20 topics assessed. A greater proportion of women discussed financial concerns ($Q = 6.50$, $p < .05$), views on sexuality (Q = 6.00, $p < .01$), feelings of anger (Q = 8.40, $p < .01$), their personal feelings (Q = 9.80, $p < .01$), and personal secrets (Q = 7.14, $p < .05$) with FR1 than with FR2 or FR3. More women discussed family problems with FR1 and FR2 than with FR3 (Q = 6.33, $p < .05$). Finally, a greater proportion of women shared problems with other friends (Q = 6.50, $p < .05$), discussed current events (Q = 6.00, $p < .05$), talked about their morals and values (Q = 6.50, $p < .05$) and shared their religious beliefs, (Q = 6.22, $p < .05$) with FR1 and FR3 than with FR2.

Equity and Close Friendships

Approximately 40% (n = 70) of the women's friendships were perceived as equitable. For the inequitable relationships (n = 104), the women perceived themselves as overbenefited in 31% (n = 32) of the friendships

TABLE 3. Percentage of Women Talking to Their Close Friends by Topic Area

Topic	All Friends (n = 182)	Two Friends (n = 41)		Three Friends (n = 16)		
		FR1	FR2	FR1	FR2	FR3
Happy Events	92.2	95.1	92.7	93.7	87.5	93.7
Sad Events	92.2	97.6	96.3	93.7	87.5	93.7
Feelings of Joy	91.8	92.7	92.7	93.7	87.5	93.7
Health Problems	90.1	97.6	95.1	87.5	75.0	68.7
Current Events	88.5	85.4	92.7	100.0	81.3	100.0
Family Problems	86.3	92.7	85.4	93.7	81.2	62.5
Mundane Details	79.1	85.4	82.9	68.7	62.5	68.7
Morals/Values	77.5	90.2	80.5	87.5	62.5	81.2
Frustrations	73.1	85.4	73.2	75.0	50.0	68.7
Feelings of Anger	64.8	70.7	63.4	75.0	43.8	50.0
Fears	64.8	75.6	58.5	68.7	43.8	50.0
Political Views	63.2	58.5	61.0	75.0	62.5	56.2
Personal Feelings	60.3	68.3	53.7	81.2	37.5	37.5
Religious Beliefs	59.3	75.6	53.7	75.0	37.5	62.5
Death/Dying	58.8	70.7	61.0	62.5	31.3	37.5
Gossip	56.6	65.9	65.9	62.5	43.8	56.2
Problems-Other Frs	44.0	53.7	39.0	50.0	25.0	43.8
Financial Concerns	39.6	51.2	36.6	31.3	12.5	6.3
Sexuality	31.9	46.3	26.8	37.5	18.8	18.8
Personal Secrets	29.3	41.5	26.8	43.7	12.5	12.5

and underbenefited in 69% (n = 72) of the friendships. When examining the reactions of women reporting on two and three close friendships, a similar overall pattern emerged: more friendships were perceived as equitable (two friends–42%; three friends–37%) or underbenefited (two friends–41%; three friends–53%) than overbenefited (two friends–17%; three friends–10%). However, when comparing the specific responses of the women reporting on two close friendships, differences in their perceptions of equity within these friendships emerged. A greater percentage of women classified their relationship with FR1 as underbenefited (48.7%) or equitable (38.5%) than as overbenefited (12.8%), whereas a greater percentage of FR2s were viewed as overbenefited (20.5%) (χ^2 = 14.75, df = 4, $p < .01$). Differences also were found for women reporting on three friendships. FR1 differed from FR2 and FR3. Specifically, a greater percentage of women perceived FR1 as underbenefited (75.0%) than either FR2 (31.0%) or FR3 (31.0%). Twenty-five percent of FR1s were equitable compared to 44.0% of both FR2s and FR3s. None of the women perceived FR1 as being overbenefited.

With respect to their personal reactions, older women who perceived their friendships as equitable and those who were underbenefited reported feeling more content and happy with their friendship than women who perceived themselves as overbenefited (F(2, 155) = 4.42, $p < .01$) (Table 4). Similarly, women who perceived their friendships as equitable and those who believed that they were underbenefited reported feeling more grateful for their friendship than women who perceived themselves as overbenefited (F(2, 147) = 10.44, $p < .001$). No significant differences were found with respect to women's feelings of anger (F(2, 144) = 1.94, $p > .05$) or guilt (F(2, 144) = .35, $p > .05$).

When examining the older women's descriptions of and feelings towards their close friends, a significantly greater percentage of women who perceived their friendships as equitable or underbenefited described their friends as "being comfortable to be with" and "someone as close as family" than women who perceived themselves as being overbenefited (χ^2 = 6.17, df = 2, $p < .05$; χ^2 = 8.91, df = 2, $p < .01$, respectively). Women who perceived themselves as being overbenefited were significantly more likely to describe their friend as some one who "makes me feel bad" than were women who perceived themselves in equitable and underbenefitting relationships (χ^2 = 13.94, df = 2, $p < .001$) (Table 4).

DISCUSSION

As is typically indicated in the friendship literature, the women in this study reported substantial social and emotional involvement with their

TABLE 4. Women's Perceptions of Equity and Reactions to Their Close Friends

Reactions	All Friends			Significance Level
	O	E	U	
Personal [Mean/(SD)]				
Happy & Content (n = 157)	3.20 (1.08)	3.70 (0.61)	3.66 (0.76)	$p < .01$
Anger (n = 147)	1.29 (0.66)	1.13 (0.33)	1.11 (0.31)	n.s.
Guilt (n = 147)	1.29 (0.71)	1.19 (0.47)	1.24 (0.51)	n.s.
Grateful (n = 150)	3.04 (1.07)	3.66 (0.59)	3.76 (0.60)	$p < .001$
Toward Friends [% Yes]				
Comfortable to Be With (n = 174)	84.4	97.1	94.4	$p < .05$
Makes Me Feel Bad (n = 174)	40.6	12.9	12.5	$p < .001$
As Close as Family (n = 174)	46.9	62.9	76.4	$p < .01$

Note: The number of friendships (n) vary due to missing data.
O = Overbenefited; E = Equitable; U = Underbenefited

close friends whereas instrumental exchanges within the friendships occurred much less frequently (e.g., Adams & Blieszner, 1989; Blieszner & Adams, 1992; Rawlins, 1992). This finding may be a function of the fact that the women and their close friends were approximately of the same age and, perhaps, facing similar health, mobility, and other physical and personal constraints. These factors may have limited the older women's opportunities and abilities to provide direct assistance. Instead, they may have relied more on social encounters and phone correspondence as a means of associating and emotionally supporting one another. Thus, although the functions of late life friendships may not be all encompassing, the "closeness" between the women and their friends allow these long-term relationships to be maintained (Johnson & Troll, 1994).

The women's social involvement with their friends included both home and community-based activities. As noted in the literature on men's friendships (cf. Nardi, 1992), sharing activities often provides the basis for the development and maintenance of friendships. These activities may have helped structure the women's social relations and provided "a forum for companionship and sociability that is socially rewarding and integrative" (Allan, 1989, p. 51).

Almost all of the women reported getting together with their close friends "just to talk." The topics of these conversations suggest that the older women disclosed a wide array of general and personal information. Yet, there also were limits to what many of the women shared, even with the closest of friends. The selectivity in subject matter may be a result of the upbringing of this cohort of women who reached adulthood prior to society's emphasis on "openness" in relationships outside of the immediate family (Lewittes, 1989; O'Connor, 1992). The women also may have been less inclined to discuss issues such as sexuality or personal secrets for fear that their friends would think they were foolish for having such thoughts and ideas "at their age" (Fisher, Reid, & Melendez, 1989). Thus, the women's personalities, their past experiences, and society's values may influence the need for and degree of disclosure and reticence within their friendships.

When exploring the instrumental, social, and affective interactions of women reporting on two and three close friends, there was greater similarities in the women's relationships with two close friends than with three friends. When differences occurred, the women consistently reported greater involvement with FR1 than FR2. Women with three close friends had more diverse patterns of interaction. This was clearly evident when examining the content of their conversations with each of these friends as significant differences resulted for half of the areas assessed. The women were the most open with FR1. Their conversations crossed all levels of information from current events to more intimate details about themselves such their personal feelings and secrets. They appeared more selective in their topics of conversations with FR2 and FR3. The rationale for and nature of these boundaries are not clearly discernable from the data available about these friendships as it is not possible to determine the specific content or level of sharing within each of the relationships. The findings do suggest, however, that within the women's network of close friends, they have a "preferred" friend with whom they most frequently turn to for intimacy and understanding.

Many of the women perceived the exchanges that occurred within their friendships as equitable. Congruent with previous studies, women who were underbenefited were just as content with their relationships as those who judged their friendships as equitable whereas women who perceived themselves as overbenefited reported less contentment (Roberto & Scott,

1986). It is interesting to note that the perceptions of equity only appeared to influence the positive feelings the women expressed about their friendships. Reports of anger or guilt about giving and receiving too little or too much from their friendships were almost non-existent among the women. Although perceiving their relationships as equitable may enhance the older women's feelings about their friendships, perceptions of inequity do not appear to result in negative feelings or major dissatisfaction with their relationships (Jones & Vaughan, 1990). Yet, the women did have a tendency to describe their friends in a more negative manner when they perceived themselves as being overbenefited. They reported that these friends sometimes made them feel bad and that they did not always feel comfortable being with them. Perhaps the women considered these occasional "outcomes" of their relationship negligible in view of the overall benefits derived from their friendship.

IMPLICATIONS FOR PRACTICE AND RESEARCH

Practice

The exchange of affective and to a lesser degree instrumental support is an important function of friendships in later life. Although the immediate obligation to reciprocate appears less salient in close friend relationships (Clark, 1984; Roberto & Scott, 1986), women in this study who perceive that they were not contributing to their friendships as much as they were gaining from them appeared less comfortable with their friends and the subsequent relationships. Formal interventions may be necessary to help older adults rethink the boundaries they place on their friendships as issues of dependency arise (Blieszner & Adams, 1992). For example, interventions may focus on such issues as self-defeating thought processes (e.g., "I cannot do anything for you") that can interfere with relationships and help the older person focus less on the comparability of exchanges and more on the importance of the total relationship to both members of the friend dyad.

Participating in social activities provided many of the women the opportunity to get together with their close friends. In some instances, this participation may contribute to and enhance the older person's psychological well-being (Cutler & Danigelis, 1993). Formal community programs, such as those offered through educational institutes, hospitals, and recreation centers need to ensure that they are designing programs that facilitate and not inhibit social interactions between attendees. Although not all older adults will be able or willing to attend such programs, practitioners interacting with elders in various domains (i.e., health care, community services) need to make a concerted effort to encourage their participation as a means of developing and maintaining friend relationships.

Research

The results of this study provide a descriptive look at the interactions of the close friendships of older women. They give us insight into close friend relationships and a more thorough understanding of the specific interactions that take place between women and close friendships in later life. Future research, employing larger and more diverse samples, is necessary to further our understanding of the complexities of close friend relationships in later life. In addition, longitudinal studies that focus on the interaction patterns of close friendships are required for a better understanding of the dynamics of relationships.

This study augments our understanding of older women's interactions with their close friends by examining multiple relationships. When researchers limit their investigations to interactions with one or two close friends, they most likely will find high similarity and solidarity within the friendships. To achieve a better understanding of the true nature of close friend relationships in later life, researchers must take a broader approach to the examination of the friendship network.

The findings of this study are limited to the perspective of one member of the friend dyad. The individual is an important source of information about the friendship, however, studying only one partner's perspective provides a bias view and denies the complexity of the relationship (Thompson & Walker, 1982). Future studies need to examine the exchange patterns of older friends from the perspective of both members of the dyad.

REFERENCES

Adams, R. (1985/86). Emotional closeness and physical distance between friends: Implications for elderly women living in age-segregated and age-integrated settings. *International Journal of Aging and Human Development, 22,* 55-75.

Adams, R. (1987). Patterns of network change: A longitudinal study of friendships of elderly women. *The Gerontologist, 27,* 222-227.

Adams, R. (1989). Conceptual and methodological issues in studying friendships of older adults. In R. Adams & R. Blieszner (Eds.), *Older adult friendships* (pp. 17-41). Newbury Park, CA: Sage.

Adams, R. & Blieszner, R. (Eds.) (1989). *Older adult friendships.* Newbury Park, CA: Sage.

Allan, G. (1989). *Friendship: Developing a sociological perspective.* Boulder, CO: Westview Press.

Armstrong, M. J., & Goldsteen, K. (1990). Friendship support patterns of older American women. *Journal of Aging Studies, 4,* 391-404.

Babchuk, N., & Anderson, T. (1989). Older widows and married women: Their intimates and confidants. *International Journal of Aging and Human Development, 28,* 21-35.

Blieszner, R., & Adams, R. (1992). *Adult friendship.* Newbury Park, CA: Sage.

Clark, M. (1984). Record keeping in two types of relationships. *Journal of Personality and Social Psychology, 47,* 549-557.

Cutler, S. N., & Danigelis, N. (1993). Organized contexts of activity. In J. Kelley (Ed.), *Activities and aging: Staying involved in later life* (pp. 146-163). Newbury Park, CA: Sage.

Dykstra, P. (1990). *Next of (non)kin: The importance of primary relationships for older adult's well-being.* Amsterdam: Swets & Zeitlinger.

Essex, M., & Nam, S. (1987). Marital status and loneliness among older women: The differential importance of close family and friends. *Journal of Marriage and the Family, 49,* 93-106.

Fehr, B. (1996). *Friendship processes.* Thousand Oaks, CA: Sage.

Fisher, C., Reid, J., & Melendez, M. (1989). Conflict in families and friendships of later life. *Family Relations, 38,* 83-89.

Goodman, C. (1985). Reciprocity among older adult peers. *Social Service Review, 59,* 269-282.

Harris, R. (1983). Pinning down the equity formula. In D. Mussick & K. Cook (Eds.), *Equity theory: Psychological and sociological perspectives* (pp. 207-242). New York: Praeger.

Johnson, C. & Troll, L. (1994). Constraints and facilitators to friendships in late late life. *The Gerontologist, 34,* 79-87.

Johnson, F., & Aries, E. (1983). The talk of women friends. *Women's Studies International Forum, 6,* 353-361.

Jones, D., & Vaughan, K. (1990). Close friendships among senior adults. *Psychology and Aging, 5,* 451-457.

Lewittes, H. (1989). Just being friends means a lot: Women, friendships, and aging. In L. Grau (Ed.), *Women in the later years: Health, social, and cultural perspectives* (pp. 139-159). New York: Harrington Park Press.

Nardi, P. (Ed.) (1992). *Men's friendships.* Newbury Park, CA: Sage.

Nussbaum, J., Thompson, T., & Robinson, J. (1989). *Communication and aging.* New York: Harper & Row.

O'Connor, P. (1992). *Friendships between women: A critical review.* New York: The Guilford Press.

Oliker, S. (1989). *Best friends and marriage: Exchange among women.* Berkeley, CA: University of California Press.

Rawlins, W. (1992). *Friendship matters: Communication, dialectics, and the life course.* New York: Aldine De Gruyter.

Roberto, K. A. (1996). Qualities of older women's friendships: Stable or volatile? *International Journal of Aging and Human Development.*

Roberto, K. A. & Scott, J. P. (1984/85). Friendship patterns of older women. *International Journal of Aging and Human Development, 19,* 1-10.

Roberto, K. A., & Scott, J. P. (1986). Equity considerations in the friendships of older adults. *Journal of Gerontology, 41,* 241-247.

Roberto, K. A., & Scott, J. P. (1987). Friendships in later life: A rural-urban comparison. *Lifestyles, 8,* 146-156.

Rook, K. (1987). Reciprocity of social exchange and social satisfaction among older women. *Journal of Personality and Social Psychology, 52,* 145-154.

Scott, J. P., & Roberto, K. (1987). Informal supports of older adults: A rural-urban comparison. *Family Relations, 36,* 444-449.

Siegel S., & Castellan, N. J. (1988). *Nonparametric statistics for the behavioral sciences* (2nd ed.). New York: McGraw-Hill.

Thompson, L. & Walker, A. (1982). The dyad as the unit of analysis: Conceptual and methodological issues. *Journal of Marriage and the Family, 44,* 889-900.

Usui, W. (1984). Homogeneity of friendship networks of older blacks and whites. *Journal of Gerontology, 39,* 350-356.

Walster, E., Walster, G., & Berscheid, E. (1978). *Equity: Theory and research.* Boston: Allyn & Bacon.

Significant Relationships Among Older Women: Cultural and Personal Constructions of Lesbianism

Dena Shenk, PhD
Elise Fullmer, PhD

SUMMARY. This paper focuses on the interactive nature of the relationship between personal and public constructions of lesbianism in the lives of older women. The cultural construction of lesbianism involves the historical and environmental context of the meaning of lesbianism framed within a societal level. Our discussion evolves around a case study of a lesbian in her eighties, living with a partner in rural Minnesota. We show that when public definitions are unavailable, older lesbians may not define certain aspects of their experience. *[Article copies available from The Haworth Document Delivery Service: 1-800-342-9678. E-mail address: getinfo@haworth.com]*

Defining oneself as a lesbian is a complex process shaped by a combination of factors that include related personal, cultural and historical

Dena Shenk is Professor and Coordinator of the Gerontology Program, University of North Carolina at Charlotte, Charlotte, NC 28223.
Elise Fullmer is Assistant Professor, Department of Sociology, Anthropology and Social Work, University of North Carolina at Charlotte, Charlotte, NC 28223.

[Haworth co-indexing entry note]: "Significant Relationships Among Older Women: Cultural and Personal Constructions of Lesbianism." Shenk, Dena and Elise Fullmer. Co-published simultaneously in the *Journal of Women & Aging* (The Haworth Press, Inc.) Vol. 8, Nos. 3/4, 1996, pp. 75-89; and: *Relationships Between Women in Later Life* (ed: Karen A. Roberto) The Haworth Press, Inc., 1996, pp. 75-89; and: *Relationships Between Women in Later Life* (ed: Karen A. Roberto) Harrington Park Press, an imprint of The Haworth Press, Inc., 1996, pp. 75-89. [Single or multiple copies of this article are available from the Haworth Document Delivery Service: 1-800-342-9678, 9:00 a.m. - 5:00 p.m. (EST). E-mail address: getinfo@haworth.com] factors. Central to this process is the eventual conscious acceptance of a lesbian identity as a part of one's self-definition. To say precisely what it means to incorporate lesbianism into one's self-definition or to live as a lesbian, however, is elusive because the term lesbian (i.e., gay woman, homosexual, bisexual) may have different meanings for different people based on their personal and culturally-based understanding of the concept.

Most studies of older lesbians discuss lesbian identity in terms of the accommodations and adaptations these women make in their day-to-day lives; that is, on social constructions and their impact on the *behavior* of individuals. Few have dealt with the relationship between public definitions and personal constructions of identity, or on the ways in which individuals seek to create understandings of whom they are in the world. One recent study discusses personal identity and public constructions within the context of the current cultural war against homosexuals (Eastland, 1995). Eastland uses Berger and Luckman's concept of "conceptual liquidation" to describe the way in which an anti-homosexual group in Oregon (the Oregon Citizen's Alliance) seeks to define lesbians and gay men out of existence and the impact of aspects of the campaign on the lives of two members of the gay community (Eastland, 1995). The framework used considers these public definitions in terms of *disempowerment,* and response of individuals in terms of *empowerment.* Empowerment as used here involves the ability of an individual (or group) to exercise free will. This ability evolves from the belief and hope that a person has control over the direction of her/his life. As pointed out by Germain and Gitterman (1987), empowerment occurs through "the creation of maximal opportunities for choice, decision making, and action consonant with age, physical and emotional states, capacities, and cultural patterns" (p. 496). Conversely, a person or group becomes disempowered when a combination of internal and external factors serves to limit opportunities for choice; thus limiting their ability to exercise free will.

In this paper, we examine the relationship between the *absence* of public definitions and personal constructions of identity in the experience of one lesbian elder, a woman in her eighties living with her partner in rural Minnesota. Our contention is that lesbian elders are unable to relate their life experience to the contemporary definitions of self available in the gay community and therefore, sometimes fail to work out a definition of the relational aspect of self. The cultural construction of the concept of lesbianism refers to the development of a definition of lesbianism within the public societal domain. The personal construction of the concept refers to the development of a definition of lesbianism within the private domain. These constructions are, of course, closely interrelated.

CULTURAL CONSTRUCTION OF LESBIANISM

The cultural construction of lesbianism involves the historical and environmental context framed within the meaning of lesbianism in the society. For older women in this culture, the context requires consideration of the understandings of homosexuality prevalent earlier in this century. Also, because the case study presented in this article is of an older *rural* woman, an understanding of the rural context is an integral part of her story.

From a North American cultural perspective, one of the most important aspects of lesbian identity is the sexual behavior of such women, which this perspective regards as abnormal. This is clearly the contention of the many conservative anti-homosexual political campaigns currently raging in this culture (Eastland, 1995). On the other hand, one can argue that lesbian identity involves more than a sexual behavior. An important question here is whether there is something uniquely different in the worldview of women whose primary sexual and/or affectional relations are with other women.

Members of this male-dominated society often defined women in terms of their relationships with men, first as daughter, and later as girlfriend or spouse. Heterosexual women have an investment in maintaining relationships with men, because they partially define their own self-identity and others know them in terms of these primary relationships with men. Women who do not have primary relationships with men as adults may be freer to create their own identities, because they cannot use the approach of formulating their self-identity based on men.

What it means to be a lesbian has varied over time and across cultures. Faderman (1981) for example, points out that in sixteenth century England, the public did not think of women as sexual beings; this allowed women to express sensuality toward one another without suspicion. In more recent times women have used the term "lesbian" to refer to political solidarity with other women. In the 1970's some feminists declared themselves "political lesbians" in their stance against patriarchy but were not necessarily involved with other women sexually (Adam, 1987). More recently, the cultural war against gay men and lesbians seeks to define homosexuality as exclusively a "behavioral choice" (Eastland, 1995). This perspective suggests that a woman chooses to "be" a lesbian and could as easily choose not to be one.

Other women, particularly older women who endured prejudice and discrimination against homosexuals in much more hostile times, may abandon terms such as lesbian or homosexual altogether in an attempt to dissociate themselves from negative stereotypes and social stigma or because they did not want to be so narrowly defined. Many of these older women carefully hid their relationships with other women and limited their contact with lesbian and gay people (Adelman, 1986; Clunis & Green, 1988). This is not particularly surprising given the cultural context within which they lived. Wolf (1980) remarks about the reality of life for the generations of homosexual women in America who are now older:

> Most of them experienced oppression, potential arrest and exposure, and an internalized view of lesbianism as a social stain. The only public place to socialize with other lesbians, if one dared risk periodic arrests, was the gay bar, though bar life was not comfortable for many women. (p. 26)

Before the 1970's only larger cities had organizations catering to lesbians. Consequently, rural women and women in smaller towns had to develop alternate ways of being in the world that did not necessarily follow patterns of women in larger urban areas. Friendship networks and social ties in rural areas often consisted of close-knit support networks and women may have had to depend on heterosexual neighbors for friendship and support. Furthermore, for most women prior to the 1970's there were also few if any role models available besides the heterosexual relationships that surrounded them. In rural communities, a strong sense of personal independence within the context of the interdependence between friends and neighbors exists. There also are guidelines and expectations for maintaining close social ties within an environment where everybody knows everyone else. These cultural values and expectations clearly affected the lives of lesbians living within that context.

The recent interest in the experience of aging in rural environments has not reversed the still overwhelming bias in the gerontological literature for urban experience (Coward, 1979), nor has it erased the major gaps that exist in our knowledge base concerning rural older adults (Lee & Lassey, 1982). It has signaled the apparent end, however, to a period where social gerontologists virtually ignored the special needs and distinctive features of aging in rural society (Coward & Lee, 1985). Little research has focused specifically on the experience of rural older women and almost no research exists on the situation of rural older lesbian women. Whereas some studies and reports include individual cases, there has been no focus on understanding or analyzing the experiences of rural older lesbian women.

We took the following case example from a research report on homeless elders. This woman, who is now in her seventies, spent most of her life living with a female partner in a rural area of Utah.

We met at age 16 in school. Our parents were farmers and we hadn't been exposed to much beyond our hometown. We were instantly attracted to each other and I don't think we spent more than a few days alone from the time we met. When my father died he left me the farm and Mary moved in a few months later. No one ever questioned us about our relationship . . . I don't think anyone particularly cared as long as we didn't talk about it openly. We didn't even talk about it much to each other . . . it just was. I had heard some about other women in Los Angeles but I couldn't relate. It was only after Mary died that I got lonely enough to sell the farm and move to Salt Lake. (Fullmer, 1987)

This case illustrates the fact that a personal definition of oneself as a lesbian is based on negotiation of personal feelings and experiences as they developed within the cultural context. Here, the *absence* of cultural understandings of the specifics of their experience has led to the absence of personal and interpersonal constructions.

PERSONAL CONSTRUCTION OF LESBIANISM

While the social definition of lesbianism focuses on sexuality, the personal definition as a lesbian is much more broadly structured with the primary emphasis on the relationship aside from the sexual aspects. There is of course, great diversity among the lifestyles and experiences of older lesbians. Our primary focus is on older lesbians who are involved in long-term committed relationships.

Kimmel (1992) has identified the three most typical family types within which lesbians grow older. These include: (a) long-term committed relationships or "companionships"; (b) social networks of friends, significant others and selected biological family members who provide mutual support of various kinds; and (c) special roles in their family of origin that reflect their unique social position. Patterns in forming intimate relationships also vary, but typically lesbians prefer a long-term committed relation with one other person (cf. Bell & Weinberg, 1978; Kehoe, 1989) and long-term committed relationships may be more common than typically assumed (Kimmel, 1992). This is not surprising, given that a committed relationship with one other person is the accepted norm in the dominant culture (Fullmer, 1995, p. 101).

Older lesbians involved in long-term committed relationships generally provide each other with a comprehensive, mutual support system and the economic advantages of sharing homes and resources (Fullmer, 1995,

p. 102). In spite of the broad nature of their interaction and mutual commitment, they may never openly acknowledge the nature of their relationship, or use the word lesbian. The cultural construction of lesbianism and the political reality of the world within which they live constrains their personal construction of the concept of lesbianism.

Adjustments to the transitions and losses that often accompany aging are different within a lesbian relationship, because of the lack of acknowledgement of the existence or the nature of the relationship between the women. If the partners, or persons significant to either person, never clearly define the relationship, others may fail to acknowledge the severity and nature of the loss. The loss of a partner in this instance may also mean the loss of material possessions or financial supports that have previously been considered joint. It might also mean that the partner may seek to hide the grieving process from others to hide the unusual character of the relationship (Fullmer, 1995).

CASE STUDY OF AN OLDER LESBIAN

This case study comes from a multi-phase research project on aging in rural Minnesota completed by the first author (Shenk) in 1986-87. Life histories were collected during the first phase of this qualitative study to gain an understanding of the worldview and categories used by the respondents. Based on this initial understanding of their lives derived from the life histories, the first author developed meaningful questions for the later phases of the project. Trained interviewers facilitated the life histories. They prompted each of the 30 respondents with the following open-ended questions:

1. Thinking about yourself and your life today, who are you? How would you describe yourself?
2. Imagine your life is a story. What would the chapters be? Tell me about them.
3. How do you get along and how do you expect your life to change in the future?

Each interview was tape-recorded and transcribed into computer files. Social network and questionnaire data were collected and are also used in the presentation of the case study. (For further discussions of the research see Shenk, 1987, 1991, 1992 and 1993; Shenk & Christiansen, 1993). The first author developed the case study based on the respondent's presentation of her life during the research process, and later correspondence with her companion.

This is the life of Maurine Strutter,[1] an 81-year old retired physical education teacher, who lived with her companion, Hilda Tretter, a retired English teacher. She described herself in the following words as she began telling her life story:

> I am a retired physical education teacher, having taught at Willmar, Minnesota for nearly 45 years–loved every minute of it. Moved out here to Clear Lake . . . but I am a native of Wisconsin–state of Wisconsin–having come to Minnesota to a college class. I'm enjoying the life out here, but I'm still looking for time to live. I keep busy, and have many, many different interests. I'm finding that the life out here is very interesting and busy, because I like the outdoors–even though I have not had time to go fishing which I like to do very much. I am . . . I like the area, I like the surroundings. I like the people and in all, I think the neighborhood has been very good to us. I just don't know how to describe myself. I tend to get a little hot-tempered sometimes, and I guess sometimes a little easy going. In other words, I can really enjoy life. I do get back to Willmar frequently, which I enjoy very much. I visit some of the former students and the parents of the students . . .
>
> As far as my health is concerned, I would say it was reasonably good. I've had a few setbacks now and then. I had pernicious anemia for which they gave me 12 shots. The doctor feels that had been very, very satisfactory and I feel that way too. I used to be a bit heavier than I was, but I'll be satisfied with what I am now. Many people have asked me whether I was German or my background. Both of my parents are foreign-born, and they came over here on their honeymoon. They didn't have enough money to go back to Germany (my mother is Polish), so here I am. They're both deceased. I have one sister who is still living in Augusta, Wisconsin. She's older than I am. And I have one brother who lived in Laramie, Wyoming. He passed away two years ago. And that's the extent of my immediate family, but I do have some nieces and nephews whom I am very fond of, and I enjoy their children very much . . .

Here Maurine describes herself in terms of her health. This is not unusual for people in her age range as they come up against lessening

---

1. Fictitious names are used to protect the anonymity of the respondent and her companion. All other details are presented as they were described during the research process.

physical abilities. She also describes herself in terms of cultural heritage, which is not unusual for second-generation Americans and is also very common in the part of the country where Maurine grew up and still lives. Furthermore, her notion of family is very traditional and she fails to include her partner, Hilda in that definition.

Maurine and Hilda live in their home overlooking Clear Lake that they have named "Birdhaven." "You know I don't live alone," she explained. "(Hilda) and I have lived here for 15 years together. We taught together in Willmar. She moved on to Rochester, but we decided to retire here." Maurine explained how they came to live in Birdhaven:

> I had this place in the woods south of here, seventy feet was given to me. A classmate of mine at La Crosse lived in Minneapolis and we were very good friends. They used to have this place. It was not the house then, it was just a summer cabin. And they used to come out here weekends, the father and mother also. Then this friend of mine died and I kind of helped her mother and father. I would clean up the place. As they became older they went to Arizona for the winter . . . So then (he) died and she was alone and it was hard for her to keep up the cabin, so she was going to sell it. They'd given me the seventy feet which I was going to build on, and as (she) was getting older, she said 'Would you take these one hundred and twenty feet?' I said, 'Only on a business proposition.' That was the only consideration. So Hilda bought this place, that's one hundred twenty feet here, and of course I had the seventy feet there–it totals two twenty altogether. We had our old cabin pulled off from here and Hilda decided to build a house.

In discussing the establishment of a retirement home, Maurine talks of circumstances rather than of interpersonal commitment. She explains that it was Hilda, her partner, who decided to build the house, making it a personal decision as opposed to a joint one. Maurine explained:

> Hilda designed this whole house. She was the architect. There are two bedrooms, both on the main level, a kitchen and (living room). We have a nice room downstairs with the TV, and we cook down there. Of course we have the bathroom up here and the shower downstairs.

In her telling of her life history, she went on to describe how they built their home:

We got our own carpenter from this area, and negotiated from the lumber yard, carpenter recommended a plumber, the Hennepin Co-op recommended an electrician, so we got going on it. And this was being built the last couple of years that I was teaching, so I came out here in the evening sometimes, every weekend, to watch the progress and check to see how things were coming along . . . But then Hilda taught at Rochester for a few years after that and then she quit. She decided that kids were getting to the point where you were almost a babysitter. And English is not an easy subject to teach . . . So she decided to retire and came out here. We both enjoy it very much. She does the things she wants to do, I do things I want to do, we do things together. She'd traveled extensively throughout Europe. She's Irish so she's spent a lot of time in Ireland, Scotland–she's part Scotch. I'm not a traveler, I'm more of a flier than she is . . .

Hilda is clearly a key person in Maurine's life and several times during the research, Maurine made comments about her relationship with Hilda. However, in these discussions Maurine seemed careful not to over-emphasize the importance of their relationship. For example, in asking about how close she is to her sister, the first author commented that Hilda was probably her closest friend. "Hilda is Scotch/Irish. We have our disagreements, but it's nothing. We always talk it out." The researcher commented that it seemed that Maurine and Hilda each had their own jobs. Maurine responded:

Yes, she does certain things and I do others. We kid each other, 'that's my department.' And we kid that one day she's boss and the next day I am . . . I don't know who is yet today. Yesterday she was. We went to St. Cloud because we had to fix up her income tax. While she did that I went to the mall and ran some errands. I forgot to take her shoes to the shoemaker, so I'll have to do that.

Maurine does the yardwork and is responsible for the cars. She told the interviewers:

Hilda doesn't like driving in the winter, so we put her car up. I have to get it started and get a tag on it. I do the driving, because she went in a ditch once and it scared her. I must be, I don't know, it happened to me, but it doesn't bother me.

Maurine loved to do woodworking and made several tables and other pieces of furniture that were in their home. Hilda does all the cooking and spends a lot of time downstairs reading and doing genealogies.

During the life history interview, the interviewer asked whether Maurine enjoyed her single life. Maurine responded: "very, very much–all the good men are gone." A graduate student who was working with these life history texts took that at face value, but the first author has always seen that as a "cover." Living in a period when society viewed homosexuality as an abnormality and particularly living in rural communities, Maurine and Hilda have lived together quietly, never saying much about their relationship to others and, we suspect, even to each other.

In recounting her life history, Maurine easily divided her story into several chapters. She outlined the chapters as: (1) family heritage, (2) childhood, (3) through high school and college, (4) travel, (5) work, (6) hobbies and (7) community involvement. She created a story of her life that incorporated her relationship with Hilda, her long-time companion, but focused on her own activities and character traits. In essence, she denied and down-played the nature of the long term commitment involved in her relationship with Hilda. Her discussions of their day-to-day activities clearly display their commitment.

They have adapted their lifestyle to the rural environment where everybody knows everyone else. In talking about their relationships with the neighbors, Maurine explained:

> We don't check on them every day or anything. We're not that kind to watch too close. Well, his car was out for two days and we were wondering. Usually he takes his car every day and she puts hers in the garage. It seems they took her car and went to the Cities overnight. So we watch, but don't want to be a bother.

A major theme that is apparent in Maurine's representation of her life is her independence. When asked how she gets along and how she expects her life to change in the future, Maurine responded:

> Well, I think I get along pretty well now. If I can find a little more time to life, as far as having things to do, I have plenty. Health is not a problem. As far as a change in life, it might be when I get to be, when I get quite a bit older, there might be a chance of moving out of here–hoping not to a rest home. In other words, I want to care for myself. I hope that will work out very well, so I don't want to be a care to anyone. In other words, I'm quite independent, I want to be independent. That's about all I can add there. Time is getting shorter and one has to face it.

In fact, the doctor diagnosed Maurine with an inoperable heart condition in 1991, and told her to curtail her activities. Hilda informed me about Maurine's death in a note:

> Maurine always spoke of you as one of her favorite people. You were mine too. Maurine is gone from us and I thought you'd like to know. Birdhaven has also gone from me and my life is changed. I'm with my sister in Northfield, two doors away. [She] lost her husband in November '93 and these two years we'll both remember. We're building for new lives of happiness together.

She enclosed two obituaries that recount Maurine's life in the following ways:

> Maurine Strutter, 87, a longtime physical education teacher in Willmar, Minn., and a member of the Minnesota Athletic Hall of Fame, died Wednesday at (a) nursing home in Willmar.
> . . . "She taught three generations of students," said her longtime friend, Hilda Tretter, of Annandale. "She was a favorite teacher. Everybody called her (nickname)."
> After retirement, Strutter moved to Annandale. She was a member of the County Historical Society and County Community Education Board and was selected the outstanding senior citizen by the Chamber of Commerce. She also directed summer recreation programs and American Red Cross swimming programs in Willmar.
> She is survived by a sister . . .

The other newspaper obituary reported very similar details, but the final paragraphs of the second include the following:

> She is survived by one sister; several nieces and nephews; and a close friend, Hilda Tretter, of Annandale.
> She was preceded in death by her parents and one brother.

I wrote and asked Hilda some questions about her relationship with Maurine and about Maurine's final illness. This was her response:

> Your letter came a long time ago, and long ago I should have written a reply. Time has passed far too quickly when I've been busy sorting, hunting and placing things in new places. Then I sit to remember, to wish and then to realize that life has to be different. I know life has to be different, and I am now picking up the happy thoughts from the past and going on . . .

The last three years of Maurine's life must have been filled with a certain anxiety. I was with her in the office when the heart specialist explained to her that she had had a serious aneurysm of the aorta and it was inoperable. She must curtail her activities—no more mowing, gardening, shoveling snow, lifting or overdoing in any way. He advised that she no longer drive her car, and that took her lifeline away. It was the hardest blow of all. She had always loved to get into her car alone to take off to one of those various meetings and all the civic things she loved to attend and do. In the time that remained for her, she never once complained of her condition, nor would she tell me how she felt physically or emotionally. She argued with me when she thought I was being overly protective—and I did try to be. I did as much of the outdoor work that she had always enjoyed, but I couldn't do it all. We hired lawn and snow work, and gradually Maurine took to sleeping more and resting on the sofa. She never did quite forgive my becoming more expert in driving her car. I'd want to take her to meetings but she'd beg off and say they'd never miss her. I know they did.

The beginning of the end came with a trip to the dentist. A tooth had to be extracted and Maurine was a bleeder. Two dentists could not stop the gushing of blood. I took her for the last time to Willmar hospital and her doctors that meant the most to her. That was the 4th of April. They did help her, stopped the bleeding and cared for her, now in a weakened condition. Finally, she moved to a nursing home in Willmar, where her friends came to call. She was alert, bright in perfect memory and conversational to the last.

I'm happy now that Maurine could have her lake home as long as she did. We knew it was no longer possible to stay here. The sale did not come until she was in the hospital; in fact, I was detained in Buffalo to close the deal a few hours after she died. I was on my way to be with her after that unhappy deal and received the call she was gone. Why I went through with that meeting, I'll never know—I was too numb to know what I was doing.

Most of the time Maurine was in Willmar, I was packing, sorting and being concerned about her. I drove every other day to be with her, the one hundred twenty miles back and forth. But this last time I did not get there. I guess it wasn't meant. Maurine was not expected to die then. Her best friend in Willmar had left her after a pleasant conversation. She was alone and slipped away from all of us. I loved her. She was my friend. She reached out to many people, and I'm happy you were one of them.

DISCUSSION

Maurine and Hilda clearly shared a significant long-term relationship. The first author never used the term lesbian in conversations and interviews with Maurine and Hilda and both authors suspect that Maurine and Hilda did not use the term between themselves. The reality is clear however; Maurine lived her life with her close friend and companion in a long-term, significant relationship. For Maurine and Hilda there was no acceptable public definition as a lesbian couple living out their lives together in rural small towns in the Midwest in the early twentieth century. With no culturally approved or sanctioned framework, they lacked a public definition upon which to formulate their own identity as a lesbian couple. They were thus disempowered by the lack of social conceptions of alternate relationships.

For Maurine and Hilda many choices were socially prescribed. Despite this, they also managed to use certain aspects of their environment to increase personal options and choices and in so doing could maintain their relationship. The rural community ethic of "minding one's own business" and looking out for each other in a non-intrusive way actually worked to the couple's advantage. It allowed them to lead their lives together without close scrutiny and potential sanctioning from others. To be accepted members of the rural community in which they lived, they had to reshape the nature of their relationship by, for example, constructing socially acceptable reasons for investing in property together and for living lives not defined by their relationship to a man, for example, the statement made by Maurine that "all the good men are gone." These personal constructions likely served, at least at some level, to subtly undermine the importance of the relationship to themselves and to the outside world. Options for this couple were limited in that they had to conform to the understandings of relationships within their environment. The lack of viable cultural definitions of lesbians disempowered them and, therefore, failed to construct a personal concept to define themselves as lesbians or an interpersonal conception of themselves as a lesbian couple.

IMPLICATIONS FOR PRACTICE AND RESEARCH

Service delivery and program design should always begin with a clear understanding of the expectations of those whom we are seeking to "serve." The attitudes and expectations of what life should be like determine the approaches of older rural lesbians to meeting their changing needs. It is difficult for many rural older women to accept care from a formal system of services because they are not comfortable with the idea of accepting help from outsiders and do not know enough about such a system to feel they can retain control (Shenk, 1987, p. 23). Their pattern of service preference also relates to the rural conception of a simple life, which does not include a formally structured, bureaucratic system governed by formal rules and guidelines. Add to that the need for women who are living a publicly unpopular lifestyle to protect their privacy and we begin to understand the challenges present in providing formal services to older rural lesbian women.

Rural older women are active manipulators of the social support system within which they meet their perceived needs and the needs of others in their social network (e.g., Shenk, 1991). Practitioners must respect the attitudes and expectations of the older women they hope to serve and be aware of the diversity that exists in the way older women structure their lives. If we treat people with respect and accorded privacy and support, we will be better prepared to meet the needs of all of the elders we serve.

There clearly needs to be more research conducted on the range of lifestyles of older lesbians and the unmet needs of older lesbians living in a range of environments. We must also begin to incorporate issues specifically related to lesbians and to older rural women into our training of service providers who work with older adults.

REFERENCES

Adam, B. D. (1987). *The rise of a gay and lesbian movement.* Boston: Twayne.

Adelman, M. (1986). *Long time passing: Lives of older lesbians.* Boston: Alyson.

Bell, A. P., & Weinberg, M. S. (1978). *Homosexualities: A study of diversity among men and women.* New York: Simon & Schuster.

Clunis, D. M., & Green, G. D. (1988). *Lesbian couples.* Seattle: Seal Press.

Coward, R. (1979). Planning community services for the rural elderly: Implications from research. *The Gerontologist, 19,* 275-282.

Coward, R., & Lee, G. (1985). *The elderly in rural society: Every fourth elder.* New York: Springer.

Eastland, L. E. (in press). The reconstruction of identity: A study of the strategies of the Oregon Citizens Alliance. In E. Berlin-Ray (Ed.), *Communication and the disenfranchised: Social health issues and implications.* Hillsdale, NJ: Erlbaum.

Faderman, L. (1981). *Surpassing the love of men.* New York: Marrow.

Fullmer, E. M. (1995). Challenging biases against families of older gays and lesbians. In G. C. Smith, S. S. Tobin, E. A. Robertson, T. Chabo, & P. W. Power (Eds.), *Strengthening aging families: Diversity in practice and policy* (pp. 99-119). Thousand Oaks, CA: Sage.

Fullmer, E. M. (1987). *Homeless elders: A group in need of services.* Report to Utah Department of Social Services, Salt Lake City, Utah.

Germain, C. B., & Gitterman, A. (1987). Ecological perspective. In A. Minahan, R. M. Becerra, S. Briar, C. J. Coulton, L. H. Ginsberg, J. G. Hopps, J. F. Longres, R. J. Patti, W. J. Reid, T. Trippodi, & S. K. Khinduka (Eds.), *Encyclopedia of Social Work* (18th ed.) (pp. 488-499). Silver Spring, MD: National Association of Social Workers.

Kehoe, M. (1989). *Lesbians over sixty speak for themselves.* New York: The Haworth Press, Inc.

Kimmel, D. C. (1992). The families of older gay men and lesbians. *Generations, 17* (3), 37-38.

Lee, G., & Lassey, M. L. (1982). The elderly. In D.A. Dillman & D.A. Hobbs (Eds.), *Rural elderly in the U.S.: Issues for the 1980's* (pp. 85-93). Boulder, CO: Westview Press.

Shenk, D. (1987). *Someone to lend a helping hand–the lives of rural older women in Central Minnesota.* St. Cloud: Central Minnesota Council on Aging.

Shenk, D. (1991). Older rural women as recipients and providers of social support. *Journal of Aging Studies, 5,* 347-358.

Shenk, D. (1992, December). *Support systems of rural older women in Denmark and Minnesota.* Paper presented at the annual meeting of the American Anthropological Association, San Francisco, CA.

Shenk, D. (1993, November). *Life's defining moments: The life history of an aging rural woman.* Paper presented at the annual meeting of the Gerontological Society of America, New Orleans.

Shenk, D., & Christiansen, K. (1993). The evolution of the system of care for the aged in Denmark. *Journal of Aging and Social Policy, 5,* 169-186.

Wolf, D. G. (1980). *The lesbian community.* Berkeley: University of California Press.

PART II:
SUPPORTIVE RELATIONSHIPS

Religious Commitment and Social Relationships: Their Relative Contributions to Self-Esteem of Catholic Sisters in Later Life

Joyce M. Mercier, PhD
Mack C. Shelley II, PhD
Edward A. Powers, PhD

SUMMARY. In this paper we examine religious commitment and social relationships of Catholic sisters and the relative contributions of these and other variables to their self-esteem in later life. Using a

Joyce M. Mercier is Professor, Department of Human Development and Family Studies, and Mack C. Shelley II is Professor, Departments of Political Science and Statistics, both at Iowa State University, Ames, IA 50011-1120.

Edward A. Powers is Associate Dean, School of Human Environmental Sciences, University of North Carolina-Greensboro, Greensboro, NC 27412-5001.

[Haworth co-indexing entry note]: "Religious Commitment and Social Relationships: Their Relative Contributions to Self-Esteem of Catholic Sisters in Later Life." Mercier, Joyce M., Mack C. Shelley II, and Edward A. Powers. Co-published simultaneously in the *Journal of Women & Aging* (The Haworth Press, Inc.) Vol. 8, Nos. 3/4, 1996, pp. 91-111; and: *Relationships Between Women in Later Life* (ed: Karen A. Roberto) The Haworth Press, Inc., 1996, pp. 91-111; and: *Relationships Between Women in Later Life* (ed: Karen A. Roberto) Harrington Park Press, an imprint of The Haworth Press, Inc., 1996, pp. 91-111. [Single or multiple copies of this article are available from the Haworth Document Delivery Service: 1-800-342-9678, 9:00 a.m. - 5:00 p.m. (EST). E-mail address: getinfo@haworth.com]

91

sample of 377 Catholic sisters with an average age of 63.5, we conducted a series of a hierarchical regression analyses to examine the
relative contributions of blocks of socio-demographic variables,
religious commitment variables, personal relationship variables, and
psychological variables to self-esteem. In the overall model, the extent to which relationships were rewarding, perceptions of themselves as women, coping strategies, and perceived self-control were
significant and thus predictive of the self-esteem of Catholic sisters.
*[Article copies available from The Haworth Document Delivery Service:
1-800-342-9678. E-mail address: getinfo@haworth.com]*

The purpose of this paper is to examine the contributions of the
religious commitment of Catholic sisters and of their personal and social
relationships to their self-esteem in later life. We also examine the influence of psychological variables on self-esteem and whether they mask or
bolster the contributions of religious commitment and personal relationships. Researchers use the concept of self-esteem to help understand the
experience of aging (Coleman, Ivani-Chalian, & Robinson, 1993). It has
been a particularly useful concept when studying how older people adjust
to changes in their lives, such as retirement or limited mobility, which may
threaten their self-perceptions and their sense of well-being. The aging
individual is increasingly vulnerable to events and conditions linked with
lowered self-esteem, including disability, poor health, loss of significant
others, and long-term change (Daniewicz, Mercier, Powers, & Flynn,
1991; Hunter, Linn, & Harris, 1981-82; Johnson, Lund, & Dimond, 1986).
Nevertheless, most studies involving self-esteem document its stability
over time (Bengtson, Reedy, & Gordon, 1985), showing neither age group
differences nor age-related changes. Thus, self-esteem is best understood
in terms of factors other than age per se (Bengtson, Cutler, Mangen, &
Marshall, 1985). In this paper, we examine three sets of variables–relationships, religious commitment, and psychological resources and self-perceptions–along with demographic variables.

SOCIAL RELATIONSHIPS AND SELF-ESTEEM

Relationships, both with family and with others, are important for self-
esteem. Coleman et al. (1993) demonstrate the prominence of ties to family
and to others for self-esteem in their longitudinal study of aging (the South-
ampton Ageing Study). While family contact was important in the initial
studies, they attribute its significant decline in importance as a source of

self-esteem in the subsequent interviews to the loss of roles in the family. Contact with persons other than family was associated with maintaining a high level of self-esteem at both waves of data collection. Contact with people other than family members emerged as the strongest predictor of high self-esteem in 1988, even stronger than the initial level in 1977-78.

Several researchers suggest that kinship interaction has little or no effect on an older person's feelings of well-being or morale (Brubaker, 1990; Lee & Elliothorpe, 1982; Lee & Ihinger-Tallman, 1980), even though family relationships are important to older people. Sibling relationships represent a continuity in family relationships that may not be present in any other form (Brubaker, 1990). Frequent contact between siblings occurs among siblings who live in close proximity (Cicirelli, 1980; Kivett, 1985; Scott, 1983). It is yet unclear what value sibling relationships have on life satisfaction or morale (Brubaker, 1990). Little, if any, research exists that shows a relationship to self-esteem of older adults, especially when looking at gender.

Lee and Shehan (1989) suggest that interactions with friends positively relate to emotional well-being. For older persons, social relations may become even more important to self-esteem after retirement. Interactions with friends have a significant positive effect on self-esteem for both sexes, regardless of employment status (Lee & Shehan, 1989). These social ties buffer the potentially negative consequences of retirement (Hatch & Bulcroft, 1992; Morgan, 1984; Thoits, 1984). In addition, friends provide important support and assistance in later life (Atchley, 1972; Roberto & Scott, 1984-85; Rosow, 1967). Friends are a valuable source of support, and are effective buffers in adjusting to role losses such as the work role and the family role (Lowenthal & Haven, 1968; Roberto & Scott, 1984-85, 1986). Blau (1981) pointed out that involvement with friends helps a person maintain a sense of usefulness and self-esteem even more effectively than do filial relationships.

Friendship may be even more important for women than for men. Szinovacz (1982) suggests that women's emotional well-being is more dependent than are men's on maintaining non-family social ties. A woman defines her identity in relation to others; her ability to make and maintain friends throughout adulthood will help her in adapting to the transitions of aging (Lenz & Myerhoff, 1985; Lewittes, 1989; Lowenthal, Thurner, & Chiriboga, 1975). Women's friendships have the power to transform and validate the self (Rose & Roades, 1987) and are more likely based on intimacy. With friends, women discuss their personal and family problems, close relationships, anxieties, and daily activities (Aries & Johnson, 1983; Rose & Roades, 1987).

SELF-ESTEEM AND CATHOLIC SISTERS

An emphasis on women and their self-esteem in later life is particularly relevant to this paper because the population being studied is a Catholic congregation of women, most of whom are in later life. Catholic sisters live as part of a community dedicated to common spiritual values that have been of overriding importance in their lives. At the time that these women joined the religious community, they believed they would experience a life of dedication to God, personal fulfillment, and lifelong security. When they entered the congregation, relationships with family and others were not considered important, and, in fact, curtailed (Quinonez & Turner, 1992). "The nurturing properties innate to the 'gentle sex' could appropriately be cultivated and expressed in ministerial contexts. Perversely, sisters were admonished constantly not to become 'attached' to others" (Quinonez & Turner, 1992, p. 90).

The changing attitude toward friendships and special ties that has occurred for Catholic sisters has been dramatic. In 1966, for example, only 32.7% of all congregations encouraged friendships, while in 1982, 79% were encouraging friendships (Neal, 1984). Today, sisters cultivate personal bonds that are viewed as an "expression of their vow to be celibate (hence, open and loving to all people)" (Quinonez & Turner, 1992, p. 90). Thus, having close friendships generally has received legitimacy in the religious congregations and the hierarchy of the church. Sisters accordingly have rearranged their lives as they interact with the larger society.

Commitment

One factor assumed not to have changed is the commitment Catholic sisters have to their church and to leading a life within a religious community. Although many women have left American Catholic sisterhoods, and the number of women entering is low, those in religious communities are dedicated and believe that they can live an apostolic life, and as such have an impact on the larger society from within the formal church structure (Deedy, 1984). Sisters are eager to be committed fully to the work of the Gospel and to those in need and without power. Each sister is an apostolic spirit that is watchful and protective of social justice (Deedy, 1984).

Faith and commitment to the church are motives for choosing sisterhood and for remaining in it. Religious commitment transforms losses in the secular world into gains and gives transcendent significance to the losses accompanying aging, because they offer those very losses in prayer for the success of the community (Magee, 1987). Magee (1987) points out that attentiveness to one's spiritual life is a decided asset to the life satisfaction of retired sisters and that it is their reason for making the lifelong commitment that they have made and carried out. Similarly, Doyle (1986) suggests that to be committed is to be involved in a relationship that has priority over alternate relationships in one's life and that the purpose of religious orders is to foster growth in commitment to Christ.

"Commitment is a key to a sense of autonomy, central to self-esteem" (Wolf, 1990, p. 201). It is an assurance for the older members that they made the right choice. Once, commitment equated self-esteem; when the option of joining a religious community provided Catholic women an attractive and esteemed alternative to the life of wife and mother (Danie-wicz et al., 1991; MacHaffie, 1986). Women entering the congregation were encouraged to develop their talents, pursue higher education, and hold administrative positions (Daniewicz et al., 1991; Ewens, 1979). Today, researchers still find evidence of a connection between religious faith and self-esteem (Forst & Healy, 1990; Wolf, 1990).

Until recently, sisters expected to do other ministries such as meditation and prayer (Mercier, Powers, & Daniewicz, 1991-92) when they could no longer function in positions for which they had trained. They viewed such commitment as part of their spirituality (Magee, 1987). Women were entering communities in great numbers before Vatican Council II, and the loss of productive work for a limited number of older sisters was no problem for the congregation. Today, the number of women entering con-gregations has declined sharply (Johns, 1987); consequently, the average age of communities is increasing (Mercier et al., 1991-92). Fewer can work to support other older sisters or to help the congregation financially in caring for the older sisters. Thus, the inability to contribute to the community may have a negative influence on self-esteem because the older sisters no longer consider themselves productive members of the community (Mercier et al., 1991-92).

Resources

Especially important for the self-esteem of older sisters should be the psychological resources they have to draw on and their self-perceptions. The sense of self-control is an important resource for older people. Exten-sive research has shown the effect of sense of control on social psycholog-ical states such as depression, anxiety, distress, life satisfaction, and well-being (Hale, Hedgepeth, & Taylor, 1985-86; Langer & Rodin, 1976; Rodin, 1987). Daniewicz et al. (1991) found that sisters who felt they were more in control of their lives scored higher in self-esteem than did sisters who experienced less control. The relationship between control and self-esteem is well established for older people (Daniewicz et al., 1991; Hunter, Linn, & Harris, 1981-82). It is not clear what this relationship will be for Catholic sisters when examined with relationship variables and religious commitment variables.

A second resource that women have to draw upon is that of coping responses. Factors reinforcing older persons' perceptions of self-efficacy are important for coping with life changing events and daily hassles (Holahan, Holahan, & Belk, 1984). Aldwin (1991) reported that relative use of coping strategies affected both perceived efficacy and depression. We expect that affective coping, that is, using emotions to cope, will have a negative effect on self-esteem, while instrumental coping, i.e., the use of information and rational processes, will have a positive effect on self-esteem (Mercier & Powers, in press). The use of instrumental coping strategies reinforces the feeling of efficacy and being able to deal with stressful situations that have arisen, while the use of affective coping strategies such as anger, hostility, and weeping vent the emotions that have built up but do nothing more.

Self-Perceptions

The perception that women have of themselves as women affects their self-esteem. For Catholic sisters, the fact that they are women was downplayed before Vatican Council II (Quinonez & Turner, 1992). The church attempted to maintain distance between Catholic sisters and other women. Little opportunity existed for the sisters to know themselves as women, much less to identify with other women and the concerns and issues of women. They hid their bodies beneath voluminous robes and covered their hair with a veil. The body was considered immaterial in a celibate life, if not dangerous (Quinonez & Turner, 1992). Sisters were not to concern themselves about their appearance or relationships with men. "The expression of emotion was frowned upon, personal relationships curtailed, sexual feelings proscribed" (Quinonez & Turner, 1992, p. 90).

Today, the situation is vastly different. Few sisters wear the habit and the veil. Dressing in "civilian" clothes and being concerned about appearance are now realities for Catholic sisters. Sisters are better able to recognize and integrate the experiences of imagination, feeling, and self-awareness within themselves (Quinonez & Turner, 1992). For all these reasons, we expect that the perceptions they hold toward themselves as women will enhance self-esteem.

In this paper, self-esteem will be regressed on blocks of religious commitment variables, relationship variables, and psychological resource and self-perception variables, in conjunction with a block of demographic control variables, to determine which set of predictors has the strongest influence on self-esteem. The statistical analysis also will assess the effect of each block in the overall model by evaluating changes in the model due to all possible combinations of blocks. This will aid in determining the robustness of each of the four sets of variables as predictors of self-esteem.

METHOD

Sample

The respondents for this study were drawn from a population of sisters in one religious community in the midwest. This is an active, working order that has had a ministry of teaching; thus many women in the congregation have high levels of education. In recent years, their ministry has changed somewhat, to more of an emphasis on working with older adults. We mailed questionnaires to each member of the congregation, excepting for those considered unable to respond. Of the 511 questionnaires mailed, 431 were returned; of those, 377 were usable. Most of the sisters who were physically able did respond. Women who did not respond or who returned incomplete questionnaires generally were older than the respondents who make up the sample. Many non-respondents were too ill to complete the questionnaire, even with assistance. These data represent 87% of the returned questionnaires and 74% of the total population.

Sisters ranged in age from 33 to 96, with a mean of 63.5 years. The women were highly educated, with modal (55%) educational attainment of a Master's degree. Fewer than 20% have a high school diploma or less. Over half the women were educators; other occupations represented include cooks, child care workers, nurses, and administrators. Thirty percent of those who responded indicated that they had a health condition, physical disability, or disability that limited their mobility. The remainder said they had no physical limitations.

Operationalization of Variables

The questionnaire, developed with the cooperation of the administrative team of the congregation, included both closed- and open-ended questions. The primary focus of the questionnaire was change, but many questions were included that examined other aspects of the sisters' lives. The dependent variable for this study is self-esteem, as measured by Rosenberg's Self-Esteem Scale (1965). The scale consists of 10 items, with a theoretical range of 10 to 50. The actual range is 17 (low self-esteem) to 50 (high self-esteem). The mean of the scale is 41.1, suggesting that generally the sisters had high levels of self-esteem. The value of the Cronbach alpha coefficient of reliability is .85. This compares favorably to the value of Ward's (1977) alpha measure of internal consistency of .74 when using this instrument on an older population.

The block of religious commitment variables includes several items measuring various aspects of commitment to the congregation. These include items asking whether the respondent would choose to be a sister again, what her reasons were for joining initially, what the advantages were of being a sister, what were the most rewarding aspects of being a sister, and to what extent religion was a rewarding part of her life. We categorized the responses to the open-ended questions and translated them into ordered categorical variables. The question about religion being a rewarding part of life was measured as a 5-point response ranging from "extremely rewarding" to "not at all rewarding." The response to the item asking whether a sister would choose to become a sister again was coded 0 "no" and 1 "yes."

The relationship variables consisted of items asking about the number of friends, the number of close friends, the existence of a confidant, whether the sister had a mentor, and a scale including four items asking how rewarding each of the following relationships was to the sisters: close friends, relationships with children, social activity groups, and family of origin. The responses to each of these items were on a 5-point range from "extremely rewarding" to "not at all." The lower end of the scale is positive and the higher end is negative. The value of Cronbach's alpha coefficient of reliability for the scale is .67. The responses to the variables measuring the numbers of close friends and numbers of friends are continuous variables. The items asking about the existence of a confidant and a mentor were coded 0 "no" and 1 "yes."

The psychological resources/perceptions block included four scales. The belief that one can control the direction of her own life is measured by items from a scale developed by Pearlin (Pearlin & Schooler, 1978; Pearlin, Lieberman, Menaghan, & Mullan, 1981). The scale consists of five items asking respondents to agree or disagree on a 5-point range to such statements as "I have little control over the things that happen to me" and "I can do just about anything I really set my mind to." The value of Cronbach's alpha coefficient of reliability is .63.

Factor analysis of the coping measure (Kahana et al., 1982) resulted in two dimensions: instrumental and affective coping. Instrumental coping includes items using rational and informational processes to cope. Affective coping includes items relating to the use of feelings such as anger, hostility, or sadness to cope. The values of the Cronbach alpha coefficients of reliability for the dimensions are .70 and .70, respectively.

The final scale in the psychological block measures respondents' perceptions of themselves as women. The scale consists of nine items asking about such things as relating to men at work, looking attractive, choosing attractive clothing, and dealing with a changing body. The 4-point response framework ranged from "not a concern" (coded 1) to "extremely concerned" (coded 4); thus the scale is coded from low (positive) to high (negative). The value of the Cronbach alpha coefficient of reliability for the scale is .79.

The demographic variables in the analysis include age (coded as actual years), highest degree earned (coded from low to high), retirement status (coded 0 "no," 1 "yes"), current living situation (ordered categorical), and limitations on mobility (coded 0 "no," 1 "yes").

RESULTS

Tables 1 and 2 summarize the results of 15 hierarchical linear regression models designed to test the robustness of each of the four sets of predictors of self-esteem. Table 1 presents the five baseline models, which measure the effects of each of the four sets of predictor variables, respectively (in Models 1 through 4), and the combined explanatory contribution of all four sets together (Model 5). The models summarized in Table 2 include all possible permutations of one or all of the four different sets of predictor variables.

By including all possible combinations of the different sets of predictor variables, we can determine readily which of the four sets of independent variables consistently are the best predictors of variation in patterns of self-esteem. Estimated standardized ordinary least squares (OLS) regression coefficients are reported. We used standardized OLS estimates to facilitate interpretation, rather than unstandardized estimates, which fail to adjust for differences in variances and measurement scale means across predictors. The dependent variable demonstrates some departure from normality, but a standard logarithmic transformation failed to improve its distributional properties noticeably. Based on that result, we decided to estimate models using the untransformed values of self-esteem, rather than to seek out more complex transformations to induce normality that would cause substantial loss of real-world interpretability. Under these circumstances, considerable protection against invalid conclusions must be sought from large-sample properties (sample sizes for these models vary

TABLE 1. Standardized Regression Coefficients, Baseline Models

Model Variable	1	2	3	4	5
Set 1: Demographics					
Limited Mobility	−.11*				−.05
Living Situation	.03	-----	-----	-----	.09
Highest Degree	.03	-----	-----	-----	−.07
Retirement Status	−.09	-----	-----	-----	.02
Age	−.09	-----	-----	-----	−.02
Set 2: Religious Commitment					
Why Join	----	−.05	-----	-----	−.10
Join Again	----	.11	-----	-----	.02
Advantages, One	----	−.11	-----	-----	.01
Advantages, Two	----	−.03	-----	-----	−.01
Advantages, Three	----	−.04	-----	-----	−.09
Lifetime Rewards, One	----	−.01	-----	-----	−.02
Commitment Rewarding	----	−.08	-----	-----	−.06
Set 3: Relationships					
Rewarding Relationships	----	-----	−.24***	-----	−.12
Confidence	----	-----	.08	-----	−.06
Number Close Friends	----	-----	.01	-----	−.01
Number Friends	----	-----	.11	-----	.07
Set 4: Psychological Resources					
Instrumental Coping	----	-----	-----	.20***	.18**
Role Perceptions	----	-----	-----	−.11*	−.16**
Affective Coping	----	-----	-----	−.17***	−.14*
Sense of Control	----	-----	-----	−.45***	−.46***
R^2	.05	.04	.09	.36	.45
Adj. R^2	.04	.01	.08	.35	.40
F	3.83	1.47	8.57	40.15	8.08
$p <$	.0022	.1799	.0000	.0000	.0000
n	350	268	333	288	215

* $p < .05$; ** $p < .01$;*** $p < .001$

from 215 to 350) and through cautious interpretation of parameter estimates having marginal significance levels (near .05).

The results for Models 1 and 2 demonstrate clearly that neither the demographic (Set 1) nor the religious commitment (Set 2) measures provide particularly good predictors of self-esteem. In these models, only limited mobility is even marginally significant ($p < .05$). Model 3 demonstrates that of the four relationship variables only the scale assessing rewarding relationship is a strongly significant predictor ($p < .001$) of

TABLE 2. Standardized Regression Coefficients, Permutations of Four Blocks of Variables

Model Variable	6	7	8	9	10	11	12	13	14	15
Set 1: Demographics										
Limited Mobility	-.15*	-.10	-.07	---	---	---	.10	-.07	-.05	---
Living Situation	.01	.03	.05	---	---	---	.02	.08	.07	---
Highest Degree	.04	.00	.00	---	---	---	.00	-.03	-.02	---
Retirement Status	-.06	-.06	-.04	---	---	---	-.02	-.03	-.01	---
Age	-.09	-.09	-.06	---	---	---	-.11	-.01	-.07	---
Set 2: Religious Commitment										
Why Join	-.04	---	---	-.09	-.09	---	-.08	-.08	---	-.10
Join Again	.09	---	---	.11	.02	---	.10	.02	---	.02
Advantages, One	-.10	---	---	-.08	.00	---	-.09	-.00	---	.02
Advantages, Two	-.00	---	---	-.04	-.02	---	-.02	-.01	---	-.02
Advantages, Three	-.06	---	---	-.03	-.07	---	-.09	-.08	---	-.09
Lifetime Rewards, One	.03	---	---	.03	-.02	---	.05	-.01	---	-.02
Commitment Rewarding	-.11	---	---	-.03	-.09	---	-.06	-.08	---	-.07
Set 3: Relationships										
Rewarding Relationships	---	-.21***	---	-.26***	---	-.14**	-.22**	---	-.12*	-.13*
Confidence	---	.07	---	-.01	---	-.01	.00	---	-.01	-.06
Number Close Friends	---	.01	---	.04	---	.04	.05	---	.03	.00
Number Friends	---	.11*	---	.17**	---	-.01	.16*	---	.01	.06
Set 4: Psychological Resources										
Instrumental Coping	---	---	.17***	---	.19**	.16**	---	.20**	.15**	.16**
Role Perceptions	---	---	-.14**	---	-.13*	-.12*	---	-.14*	-.14**	-.15*
Affective Coping	---	---	-.19***	---	-.15*	-.16**	---	-.15*	-.19***	-.14*
Sense of Control	---	---	-.42***	---	-.47***	-.44***	---	-.45***	-.42***	-.46***
R^2	.10	.13	.38	.15	.40	.40	.18	.41	.41	.44
Adj. R^2	.05	.10	.36	.11	.37	.38	.13	.36	.38	.40
F	2.24	5.24	18.53	3.93	12.71	22.46	3.26	8.97	14.03	10.52
p-value	.0107	.0000	.0000	.0000	.0000	.0000	.0000	.0000	.0000	.0000
n	267	329	285	254	224	278	253	223	275	216

* $p < .05$; ** $p < .01$; *** $p < .001$

self-esteem. The four relationship measures account collectively for less than 9% of total variation in self-esteem. In sharp contrast, the psychological variables included in Model 4 perform much better and the partial effects of each of the four variables in Set 4 are significant individually.

The strength of the control scale is particularly notable. Model 5, in which we include all twenty predictors jointly, shows that the strong partial effect of the control scale, a psychological variable, persists. Also, compared to the results for Models 1 through 4, in Model 5 the significance of the scale assessing the sisters' perceptions of themselves as women is heightened noticeably, the effect of the rewarding relationships scale is attenuated to the point of nonsignificance, and the significance of two psychological measures–instrumental coping and affective coping–diminishes somewhat but remains potent. The full model (Model 5) explains an impressive (for cross-sectional data) 45.5% of variation in self-esteem (or 39.8%, by the adjusted R^2 measure), although both this noticeable discrepancy between the two measures of explained variation and the much more marked attenuation of F-ratios between Model 4 (F = 40.15) and Model 5 (F = 8.08) attest to the relative inefficiency of the "full" Model 5, which includes a large number of nonsignificant variables.

The key findings of Models 6 through 15, shown in Table 2, are summarized fairly quickly by examining the attained significance levels for the various predictors. What one looks for in such a comparison of permuted model structures principally is evidence of attenuation–that is, reduced values of the estimated standardized OLS parameters–or suppression–that is, the contrary pattern of heightened coefficient values and lower levels of attained significance. With some fluctuation, which is to be expected due to sampling variation and differing patterns of collinearity among the different permuted combined sets of predictors, the previously reported results generally persist across Models 6 through 15. That is, variables that were significant predictors in Models 1 through 5 remain significant in these latter models, although there is some fluctuation in their estimated values and therefore in their levels of significance. The only case of a predictor that was not statistically significant in any of Models 1 through 5 becoming even marginally significant in any of Models 6 through 15 is number of friends, in Models 7, 9, and 12 (and only in Model 9 is its effect significant at $p < .01$). With that exception, the predictors that were nonsignificant in Models 1 through 5 remained so in subsequent models. Limited mobility, which was significant when it appeared in Model 1 with only other demographic predictors and which became nonsignificant in the presence of all other predictors in the "full" model (Model 5), is somewhat erratic in the remaining models; it is significant in Model 6, when religious commitment variables are added to the demographics, but not for any other permutation of predictor variable sets.

The most consistent findings from a comparison across the models in Tables 1 and 2 are that the following variables are significant under all alternate model specifications: instrumental coping, perceptions of themselves as women, affective coping, and control. In addition, rewarding relationships was significant in every instance except the full model (Model 5), where collinearity with other measures increased its p-value above .05. Of these, by far the strongest consistent effects, as measured by the size of the standardized OLS parameter estimates, are for control. Four of the five consistently significant variables are the psychological measures contained in Set 4. The relevance of the psychological constructs is emphasized most dramatically when noting that R^2 and adjusted R^2 values become impressive (i.e., exceed 35% of explained variation) only when the four psychological measures are included in any model. The three other sets of predictors combined can muster an R^2 value of only about .18 (in Model 12, in which only rewarding relationships and number of friends are significant predictors). Adding the set of psychological variables to any other single set or combined sets of independent variables invariably increases R^2 to at least .35. The only exception to this dominance of the psychological predictors is the rewarding relationships variable, which was drawn from the relationship variables of Set 3.

We also analyzed the data using several model-building strategies–forward selection, backward elimination, and stepwise modeling–designed to locate an "optimal" combination of predictor variables (results not shown due to space constraints). Two of these techniques–forward selection and stepwise modeling–converge to the same solution, with the following significant ($p < .05$) predictors: control, affective coping, instrumental coping, perceptions of themselves as women, and rewarding relationships. The key conclusion from these results is to reinforce the previous finding that rewarding relationships is the only exogenous variable apart from the set of psychological variables to be a significant predictor of self-esteem. A slightly different result emerges from the backward elimination regression; in addition to the five variables that were significant in the forward and stepwise procedures, reason for joining and current living situation also were significant.

Finally, we conducted partial-F tests to ascertain the relevance of each set of predictor variables within the full model (Model 5). These results show the relative importance of each of the four sets of explanatory variables within the overall analysis. Neither Set 1 (demographics) (F = 1.26, p = .2844) nor Set 2 (religious commitment) (F = 1.92, p = .0680) is significant by this assessment. However, given the focus of this paper on the contribution of relationships to self-esteem, it is important to note that both Set 3 (relationships) (F = 6.13, p < .0001) and Set 4 (psychological variables) (F = 23.51, p < .0001) are significant. These results add yet more strength to our previous conclusions that the contributions of relationships and psychological measures both are essential to understanding patterns of self-esteem among women in later life.

DISCUSSION

When viewed alone, the set of religious commitment variables contributes almost nothing to self-esteem. In fact, the model in which self-esteem is regressed on the religious commitment variables is the only model that does not have a significant F-value. None of the religious commitment variables contributes significantly to self-esteem. Two variables approach significance at the p < .07 and p < .08 levels: an item asking whether a sister would choose to be a sister again and an item looking at the advantages of being a sister, respectively. Because the literature shows a relationship between religious commitment and self-esteem (Forst & Healy, 1990; Wolf, 1990), it is surprising that this pattern did not emerge here. In all of the analyses conducted, neither the demographic nor the religious commitment sets of variables made significant contributions to self-esteem. One questions whether it might be the declining memberships of the congregations and a resultant anxiety about the future that is having an effect here. We suggest that the sisters are affected by the lack of new members and the crisis of old age that is occurring in the community. Even though their commitment is strong and their spirituality significant, the security of the community, with fewer revenue-producing members and more retired members who require increasing shares of resources, may be causing the sisters concerns about what lies ahead.

On the other hand, the set of variables for relationships does include a strongly significant variable, i.e., the rewarding relationships scale. Rewarding relationships significantly affect self-esteem in every model, except for the full model. It is hard to explain why this variable is not significant in the full model; it approaches significance, but has been attenuated considerably in this model compared to the other models. As mentioned before, another variable or combination of variables must be interacting with rewarding relationships and suppressing it in the full model. However, in the subsequent analyses, rewarding relationships maintains its position as the only exogenous variable other than the four psychological variables to predict self-esteem. When partial-F tests were conducted, the set of relationship variables contributed significantly to self-esteem.

It is easy to understand why relationships should be significant. The literature provides strong documentation for the fact that for older women, relationships are important to self-esteem (Lee & Shehan, 1989; Roberto & Scott, 1984-85; Rose & Roades, 1987). When retirement is part of that picture, relationships appear to become even more important (Hatch & Bulcroft, 1992; Morgan, 1984; Thoits, 1984). The rewarding relationships scale consists of items examining how rewarding certain relationships are (i.e., close friends, relationships with children, social activity groups, and family of origin). For these Catholic sisters, having close friends, relationships with children, being active socially in various groups, and interacting with their families is very rewarding and positively related to self-esteem (Lee & Shehan, 1989). The non-family contacts suggested by the scale are considered more important for women than for men in influencing self-esteem (Szinovacz, 1982). The findings of this study support those of Coleman et al. (1993), who report that "others" and "family" are sources of self-esteem and that these sources significantly relate to self-esteem in later life.

It is particularly important to note how meaningful these relationships are to Catholic sisters when one reflects on the history of many of the Catholic congregations, when the women were expected to "curtail" relationships with families of origin and with friends whom they had prior to entering the community (Quinonez & Turner, 1992). The earlier exhortation not to become "attached" to others evidently has not prevented the sisters from developing attachments once they were acceptable. The ability to interact freely with friends and relatives has influenced the self-esteem of the sisters. As Blau (1981) suggested, involvement in a friend relationship influences a person's sense of usefulness and self-esteem. This consideration also seems particularly appropriate considering the more recent statement that cultivating personal bonds is an expression of vows of celibacy for the sisters that allow them to be open and loving to *all* people (Quinonez & Turner, 1992).

The psychological and perception variables of control, coping, and perception of self as a woman all related to their self-esteem. The strength of these variables was maintained regardless of what other variables were in the model. Sense of control is particularly strong in this study. It is an important resource for older people in general, and, more specifically, for older women (Hale, Hedgepeth, & Taylor, 1985-86; Langer & Rodin, 1976; Rodin, 1987). For women who entered the Catholic congregations when they were young and for whom that commitment meant sacrificing other aspects of their lives such as the roles of wife and mother, a sense of control over at least part of their lives is necessary. Daniewicz et al. (1991) reported that sisters who indicated a high degree of control over their lives also exhibited high esteem, and that this high level of control did not negate or replace their religious commitment to the vows that they had taken.

Both instrumental and affective coping related to self-esteem. Instrumental coping was positively related (i.e., the more use of rational and informational types of coping, the higher the self-esteem), while affective coping, or using the expression of feelings to cope, was negatively related to self-esteem. The more a sister used weeping, hostility, or anger to cope, the lower was her self-esteem (Mercier & Powers, in press). This finding is also supported by Aldwin (1991), who reported that the relative use of coping strategies affected both perceived efficacy and depression.

It is noteworthy that the scale assessing the sisters' perceptions of themselves as women had a positive effect on self-esteem. The more positive the perceptions, the higher the sisters' level of self-esteem. This relationship held up throughout all the models that included the psychological/perception set of predictor variables. If the sisters were not concerned about such things as relating to men at work, looking attractive, choosing attractive clothing, and dealing with a changing body, their self-esteem was higher. This only makes sense. If someone–anyone–is overly concerned about how she looks and how she is relating to others or how she perceives her role as a woman, it is going to affect her sense of well-being as well as the way she approaches her job, or in this case, her ministry. She will become too self-conscious to relate effectively to anyone, and her self-esteem will be affected. Since sisters hid their bodies under voluminous robes and their hair under veils up until the time of Vatican II, they have managed to handle these changes admirably. As Quinonez and Turner (1992) argued, the sisters have become better able to recognize and integrate the experiences of imagination, feeling, and self-awareness within themselves.

It is apparent, in looking at all the analyses and the consistency of the findings throughout, that the contributions of both relationships and psychological/perception measures are fundamental to understanding patterns of self-esteem among women in later life. More specifically, the results of this study show that both relationships and psychological and perception measures are keys to understanding patterns of self-esteem among Catholic sisters in later life, while religious commitment has little impact.

CONCLUSIONS

What conclusions can be drawn from this study? First, it is important to examine the strength of the five variables that dominate this analysis:

rewarding relationships, control, instrumental coping, affective coping, and the sisters' perceptions of themselves as women. These variables maintained their strength throughout the analysis, regardless of other variables included in alternative models. These are variables that the literature reports are important to the self-esteem of older persons, and to women in particular. What is notable here is that these variables are also important to the self-esteem of a congregation of Catholic sisters whom some might say are atypical of the general aging population.

Are these women atypical, or are they typical of the new group of highly-educated career women who may or may not marry, but who, even if they do marry, may be single before they reach retirement? For these sisters, aging brings decreased mobility and decreased control over their lives and some uncertainty for what lies in their future. Older sisters have lower self-esteem than do younger sisters. In fact, when we entered only the demographic variables into the model with self-esteem, limited mobility was significantly related to self-esteem. (This effect disappeared when the sets of relationship variables and/or the psychological/perception variables were entered.) This outcome is consistent with what is true for older women in general. Limited mobility affects the self-esteem of older people, but when such variables as psychological resources and social support are available, the impact of limited mobility becomes much less.

Relationships are important to all women. Friends and family offer support and encouragement. They buffer change and loss and help maintain self-esteem. Relationships, or social resources, play an important role in the self-esteem of older women, as do psychological resources—especially a personal sense of control. Control over one's situation and the influence of control on self-esteem are well-established in the general population. Control for a Catholic sister is important in spite of the fact that she had taken vows of obedience when she entered the community. Although the sister has received more autonomy and decision-making power because of Vatican II, it is important to recognize that obedience to the authority of the order and of the Church are still important components of her commitment (Daniewicz et al., 1991).

IMPLICATIONS FOR PRACTICE AND RESEARCH

Having certain psychological/perception and social resources such as coping abilities, a sense of control, a positive perception of self as a woman, and friends and family are all essential to the self-esteem of these sisters and to all older women. For Catholic sisters, in particular, it is important to provide support for building and maintaining friendships both within and beyond the congregation. Allowing and encouraging friendships that exist within and outside the congregations may be especially important for the oldest sisters, who may have had that option in their repertoire for a relatively short time. Such encouragement may be especially important because elder sisters may not have maintained the strong family ties that other older people have, given the constraints they were under when they entered their congregation. Providing opportunities to meet with family and friends outside the congregation may be one way of helping them to strengthen those bonds.

Helping the sisters develop a stronger perception of themselves as women may also increase their feelings of self-esteem and provide opportunities for the oldest sisters to retain a sense of control over their own bodies and lives. Programs that are set up within the congregations may help the older women to realize their own strengths and to renew some skills such as coping strategies and assertiveness that they possess. Such programs in the larger community provide encouragement for older women to develop and maintain their personal resources, to avoid unnecessary intervention, and to remain as independent as possible.

Future research into the friendship patterns that Catholic sisters have developed may be helpful in understanding the processes that older women generally must develop to broaden their social networks. A more in-depth examination of the social and psychological resources that Catholic sisters have and how these relate to self-esteem and successful aging of these earlier career women will facilitate that process. As women age and frequently outlive their contemporary family members, they need to be encouraged to continue to allow their social networks to expand rather than shrink. Studying women once exhorted not to develop those resources when they were young and who since gained that freedom and encouragement may help us to understand far more about that process than by studying women who have been developing such bonds for a lifetime. Catholic sisters, in effect, can provide us with a laboratory to help women in general who are busily engaged in succeeding in a career, and perhaps disregarding other aspects of their lives.

REFERENCES

Aldwin, C. M. (1991). Does age affect the stress and coping process? Implications of age differences in perceived control. *Journal of Gerontology: Psychological Sciences, 46,* P174-P180.

Aries, E. J., & Johnson, F. L. (1983). Close friendship in adulthood: Conversational content between same-sex friends. *Sex Roles, 9,* 1183-1196.

Atchley, R. C. (1972). *The social forces in late life.* Belmont, CA: Wadsworth Publishing Company.

Bengtson, V. L., Cutler, N. E., Mangen, D. J., & Marshall, V. W. (1985). Generations, cohorts, and relations between age groups. In R. H. Binstock, & E. Shanas (Eds.), *Handbook of aging and the social sciences* (pp. 304-338). New York: Van Nostrand Reinhold.

Bengtson, V. L., Reedy, M. N., & Gordon, C. (1985). Aging and self conceptions: Personality processes and social contexts. In J. E. Birren & W. Schaie (Eds.), *Handbook of the psychology of aging* (2nd ed.) (pp. 544-593). New York: Van Nostrand Reinhold.

Blau, Z. S. (1981). *Aging in a changing society.* (2nd ed.). New York: Franklin Watts.

Brubaker, T. (1990). Families in later life: A burgeoning research area. *Journal of Marriage and the Family, 52,* 959-981.

Cicirelli, V. G. (1980). Sibling relationships in adulthood: A life span perspective. In L. W. Poon (Ed.), *Aging in the 1980's* (pp. 455-462). Washington, DC: American Psychological Association.

Coleman, P. G., Ivani-Chalian, C., & Robinson, M. (1993). Self-esteem and its sources: Stability and change in later life. *Ageing and Society, 13,* 171-192.

Daniewicz, S. C., Mercier, J. M., Powers, E. A., & Flynn, D. (1991). Change, resources and self-esteem in a community of women religious. *Journal of Women & Aging, 3,* 71-91.

Deedy, J. (1984). Beyond the convent wall: Sisters in the modern world. *Theology Today, 40,* 421-425.

Doyle, J. C. (1986). Commitment in a religious order: A sociological view. *Review for Religious, 2,* 188-204.

Ewens, M. (1979). Removing the veil: The liberated American nun. In R. Ruether & E. McLaughlin (Eds.), *Women of spirit: Female leadership in Jewish and Christian traditions* (pp. 255-278). New York: Simon and Schuster.

Forst, E., Jr., & Healy, R. M. (1990). Relationship between self-esteem and religious faith. *Psychological Reports, 67,* 378.

Hale, W. D., Hedgepeth, B. E., & Taylor, E. B. (1985-86). Locus of control and psychological distress among the aged. *International Journal of Aging and Human Development, 21,* 1-8.

Hatch, L. R., & Bulcroft, K. (1992). Contact with friends in later life: Disentangling the effects of gender and marital status. *Journal of Marriage and the Family, 54,* 222-232.

Holahan, C. K., Holahan, C. J., & Belk, S. S. (1984). Adjustment to aging: The role of life stress, hassles, and self-efficacy. *Health Psychology, 3,* 315-328.

Hunter, K. I., Linn, M. W., & Harris, R. (1981-82). Characteristics of high and low self-esteem in the elderly. *International Journal of Aging and Human Development, 14,* 117-125.

Johns, B. (1987). *Promises to keep: Tri-conference retirement project.* United States Catholic Charities.

Johnson, R. J., Lund, D. A., & Dimond, M. F. (1986). Stress, self-esteem and coping during bereavement among the elderly. *Social Psychological Quarterly, 49*, 273-279.

Kahana, E., Fairchild, T., & Kahana, B. (1982). Adaptation. In D. J. Mangen & W. A. Peterson (Eds.), *Research instruments in social gerontology: Vol. 1: Clinical and social psychology* (pp. 145-193). Minneapolis: University of Minnesota Press.

Kivett, V. (1985). Consanguinity and kin level: Their relative importance to the helping network of older adults. *Journal of Gerontology, 40*, 228-234.

Langer, E. J., & Rodin, J. (1976). The effects of choice and enhanced personal responsibility for the aged: A field experiment in an institutional setting. *Journal of Personality and Social Psychology, 34*, 191-198.

Lee, G., & Elliothorpe, E. (1982). Intergenerational exchange and subjective well-being among the elderly. *Journal of Marriage and the Family, 44*, 217-224.

Lee, G., & Ihinger-Tallman, M. (1980). Sibling interaction and morale: The effects of family relations on older persons. *Research on Aging, 2*, 367-391.

Lee, G., & Shehan, C. L. (1989). Social relations and the self-esteem of older persons. *Research on Aging, 11*, 427-442.

Lenz, E., & Myerhoff, B. (1985). *The feminization of America.* Los Angeles: Jeremy P. Tarcher, Inc.

Lewittes, H. J. (1989). Just being friendly means a lot–Women, friendship and aging. In L. Grau (Ed.) *Women in the later years* (pp. 139-160). New York: The Haworth Press, Inc.

Lowenthal, M. F., & Haven, C. (1968). Interaction and adaptation: Intimacy as a critical variable. *American Sociological Review, 33*, 20-31.

Lowenthal, M. F., Thurner, M., & Chiriboga, D. (1975). *Four stages of life.* San Francisco, CA: Jossey-Bass.

Magee, J. J. (1987). Determining the predictors of life satisfaction among retired nuns: Report from a pilot project. *Journal of Religion and Aging, 4(1)*, 39-49.

MacHaffie, B. J. (1986). *Her story: Women in the Christian tradition.* Philadelphia: Fortress Press.

Mercier, J. M., Powers, E. A., & Daniewicz, S. C. (1991-92). Aging Catholic sisters' adjustment to retirement. *Journal of Religious Gerontology, 8*, 27-39.

Mercier, J. M., & Powers, E. A. (in press). Sense of control among women religious. *Journal of Religious Gerontology.*

Morgan, L. A. (1984). Structural determinants of men's and women's personal networks. *Journal of Marriage and the Family, 46*, 323-331.

Neal, M. A. (1984). *Catholic sisters in transition: From the 1960's to the 1980's.* Wilmington, DE: Michael Glazier, Inc.

O'Bryant, S. L. (1988). Sibling support and older widows' well-being. *Journal of Marriage and the Family, 50*, 173-183.

Pearlin, L. I., Lieberman, M. A., Menaghan, E. & Mullan, J. T. (1981). The stress process. *Journal of Health and Social Behavior, 22*, 337-356.

Pearlin, L. I., & Schooler, C. (1978). The structure of coping. *Journal of Health and Social Behavior, 19*, 2-21.

Quinonez, L. A., & Turner, M. D. (1992). *American Catholic sisters*. Philadelphia: Temple University Press.

Roberto, K. A., & Scott, J. P. (1984-85). Friendship patterns among older women. *International Journal of Aging and Human Development, 19,* 1-11.

Roberto, K. A., & Scott, J. P. (1986). Equity considerations in the friendships of older adults. *Journal of Gerontology, 41,* 241-247.

Rodin, J. (1987, October). *The determinants of successful aging*. Presented as a Science and Policy Seminar, The Federation of Behavioral, Psychological and Cognitive Sciences, Washington, D.C.

Rosenberg, M. (1965). *Society and the adolescent self-image*. Princeton, N. J.: Princeton University Press.

Rose, S., & Roades, L. (1987). Feminism and women's friendships. *Psychology of Women Quarterly, 11,* 243-254.

Rosow, J. (1967). *Social integration of the aged*. New York: Free Press.

Scott, J. P. (1983). Siblings and other kin. In T. H. Brubaker (Ed.), *Family relationships in later life* (pp. 47-62). Beverly Hills, CA: Sage.

Szinovacz, M. (1982). Introduction: Research on women's retirement. In M. Szinovacz (Ed.), *Women's retirement: Policy implications for recent research* (pp. 13-21). Beverly Hills, CA: Sage.

Thoits, P. (1984). Explaining distributions of psychological vulnerability: Lack of social support in the face of stress. *Social Forces, 63,* 453-481.

Ward, R. A. (1977). The impact of subjective age and stigma on older persons. *Journal of Gerontology, 32,* 227-232.

Wolf, M. A. (1990). The call to vocation: Life histories of elderly women religious. *International Journal of Aging and Human Development, 31,* 197-203.

Female Farm Operators:
Attitudes About Social Support
in Their Retirement Years

M. Jean Turner, PhD

SUMMARY. In a traditionally patriarchal occupation, women farm operators may be particularly at risk of inadequate planning and support in later years. This study examined the acceptability of a set of in-home and live-in social support options potentially available to 151 women farm operators. For the married women, help from a spouse was most acceptable. The only other option rated as very acceptable by many of the women was having a child come by to help. The study also examined factors differentiating between women who indicated a particular social support option as acceptable and those who did not. Few of the demographic or attitude variables distinguished between the groups. The discussion concludes with recommendations for future research and with the practice implications of the findings. *[Article copies available from The Haworth Document Delivery Service: 1-800-342-9678. E-mail address: getinfo@haworth.com]*

Female farm operators comprise a unique group of aging women. These women have frequently been "invisible" in studies of farm opera-

M. Jean Turner is Assistant Professor, School of Human Environmental Sciences, College of Agricultural, Food, and Life Sciences, University of Arkansas, Fayetteville, AR 72703.

This research supported by the National Research Initiative Competition Grants Program, USDA, "Retirement Preparation of Farm Families: Planning for Well-Being in Later Life." Award # 93-37401-9047.

[Haworth co-indexing entry note]: "Female Farm Operators: Attitudes About Social Support in Their Retirement Years." Turner, M. Jean. Co-published simultaneously in the *Journal of Women & Aging* (The Haworth Press, Inc.) Vol. 8, Nos. 3/4, 1996, pp. 113-127; and: *Relationships Between Women in Later Life* (ed: Karen A. Roberto) The Haworth Press, Inc., 1996, pp. 113-127; and: *Relationships Between Women in Later Life* (ed: Karen A. Roberto) Harrington Park Press, an imprint of The Haworth Press, Inc., 1996, pp. 113-127. [Single or multiple copies of this article are available from the Haworth Document Delivery Service: 1-800-342-9678, 9:00 a.m. - 5:00 p.m. (EST). E-mail address: getinfo@haworth.com]

113

tors and rarely examined as a special population of women (Kalbacher, 1983; Leckie, 1993; Sachs, 1983). Yet, understanding this growing number of nontraditional women in an occupation that has steadfastly held to more traditional gender role distributions of labor (Gallagher & Delworth, 1993; Gasson & Winter, 1992) has important implications for understanding aging women and their social support needs.

Because retirement affects each individual differently, partly due to unique life experiences, female farm operators' retirement transition should differ from that of women who do not own their own business. These women are breaking gender barriers in a continuing patriarchal establishment, the family farm (Leckie, 1993; Sachs, 1983). In so doing, their life experiences differ from other women in more traditionally female occupations and from male farm operators. Understanding the acceptability of a variety of informal social support sources available to female farm operators can provide important insights into the expected support systems of a growing number of nontraditional women.

Preparing for the retirement transition and the changes that follow requires consideration of many dimensions such as physical health, life satisfaction, and family relationships. Researchers repeatedly report that, on the average, people fail to plan adequately for later life (Bailey & Turner, 1994; Kragie, Gerstein, & Lichtman, 1989). Farm operators are especially vulnerable to a lack of planning for later years (Turner, 1993) because of a belief that they will never retire but rather will "die on the tractor." If they think about retirement at all, they believe the land will take care of them, a belief that may no longer be true considering the changing nature of the family farm. When planning does occur, the focus is often on ensuring economic stability through financial planning activities such as making a will, estate planning, and establishing savings (Bailey & Turner, 1994). As a result, women farm operators may overlook several key components of the retirement planning process.

The examination of one's social support network must be a part of the total retirement planning process. Receiving positive informal social support has been associated with continued quality of life in later years (Kramer, 1991). However, individuals rarely include an assessment of one's informal social support as a part of comprehensive planning for retirement. Older adults often assume that family or friends will provide the necessary support, regardless of prior communication about expectations. The mythology of farm life, as providing a readily available support system for aging farmers, contributes to this lack of planning by farm operators of both genders. The changing demographics of farm families, combined with expanding occupational choices for farm children, may place this special population of women at risk of increasing isolation as they age.

The number of female farm operators is rising (Kalbacher, 1985; U.S. Bureau of the Census, 1993). They are generally much older than their male counterparts (Kalbacher, 1983). This suggests that a growing number of farm women are beginning to face the transition into retirement or to deal with health problems that may require assistance from their social support networks. Counselors, educators, Cooperative Extension agents, and other professionals working with female farm operators must make every effort to ensure that these women are adequately prepared for later life on or off the farm.

LITERATURE REVIEW

Theoretical Perspective

The "substitution model" best explains the use of informal support by older adults (Scott & Roberto, 1985, p. 624). According to the substitution model, when elders need help they initially depend upon family members. When the family is not able to provide the needed support, older adults will look to other informal supports such as friends or neighbors. When older adults perceive that informal options are not available, they then turn to formal support systems for assistance (Shanas, 1979).

The substitution model is especially useful when studying a distinct population such as farm women. The basic principle of this theoretical model is the expectation that family members will be available to provide support if health fails in later life (Scott & Roberto, 1985). The myth of the farm family assumes that strong family ties exist, ensuring that, when needed, older family members will have adequate support. However, female farm operators may be especially vulnerable to a lack of support in later life because of this assumption. The farming population may also be more at risk of a lack of formal support due to its rural location (Mercier, Paulson, & Morris, 1988). Rural residents, especially those living on farms, generally have very limited formal support programs available when needed to supplement informal support because of distance from town, lack of population density, and limitations of financial resources with which to provide rural formal services.

Informal Social Support

Older adults must consider their informal social network as an important factor in planning for later years. Although many farmers do not plan to retire, health problems can lead to the need for support in later years to continue independent living. Family members supply most of this informal social support (Dwyer, Lee, & Coward, 1990; Shanas, 1979). When available, most older adults prefer support from family members to that of non-family members (Krause, 1990; Peters, Hoyt, Babchuk, Kaiser, & Iijima, 1987; Pilisuk & Parks, 1988; Shanas, 1979; Stoller & Pugliesi, 1988). Friends and neighbors are also a vital part of the informal support network, especially in rural areas. However, research has shown that friends and neighbors do not fill the void created if family members are not able or present to provide assistance (Peters et al., 1987). Estimates suggest that without the presence of informal support, as many as 10% of the older adults now living independently would have to be placed in nursing homes (Cantor, 1983; Kosberg & Cairl, 1986).

Scott and Roberto (1985) studied 571 rural elderly poor living in West Texas. Their sample members reported using informal support networks more often than formal support networks. When the respondents relied on formal support, they used it in combination with, not separate from, informal support (Scott & Roberto, 1985). In a study of 1,136 elderly adults in Cleveland, Ohio, Krause (1990) found that urban elders in need of help also used informal support more often than formal support.

Antonucci and Akiyama (1987) found differences between the informal social support networks as a result of gender. In their study of 214 men and 166 women ranging from 50 to 95 years of age, the men most often gave help to and received help from their spouses. The women reported that they gave and received help from people other than their spouses such as children or friends (Antonucci & Akiyama, 1987).

Farm Life

Beyond being a physical system affecting the earth, agriculture is also a social system (Leckie, 1993). Throughout history, despite the many contributions of women in agricultural production, this social system has been patriarchal in nature (Sachs, 1983). Thus, men often overlook and minimize women's roles in agriculture and contributions to the well-being of rural communities (Geisler, Waters, & Eadie, 1985; Kalbacher, 1985; Kivett, 1990; Leckie, 1993; Sachs, 1983). The indistinguishable nature of work and family on the family farm, both physically and psychologically, also has contributed to difficulty in discerning women's actual involvement in farm work (Rosenfeld, 1985). These factors have added to the invisibility of women farmers. However, the rising number of reported female farm operators combined with improved methods of data collection have provided an opportunity to more clearly examine this group of aging women and their social support systems as they prepare for their retirement years.

The number of family farms has been in decline since its peak in 1935 (Kalbacher, 1983). Simultaneously, the number of female operated family farms has increased (Kalbacher, 1983, 1985; Leckie, 1993; U. S. Bureau of Census, 1992). In 1950, females operated only 2.7% of all farms compared to 5.0% in 1970 (Kalbacher, 1983, 1985) and to 7.5% in 1992 (U. S. Bureau of Census, 1994). The agricultural establishment has been slow to recognize these gender changes in farm ownership.

The 1978 Census of Agriculture and the 1979 Farm Finance Survey were the first attempts to gain detailed information about farm characteristics by gender (Kalbacher, 1985). Female operators, with an average age of 57.6 years, are older than their male counterparts, averaging 52.9 years of age. Over one-quarter of the women operators are over the age of 70 years compared to 11% of the men. Most of the women operators live on the farm and do not have significant paid employment away from the farm. They have lived an average of 18.4 years on the land they currently farm. Their farms are generally smaller and provide less income than that of male farmers. Approximately 50% of the female farmers operate farms in the southern region compared to only 25% in the north central region (Kalbacher, 1983, 1985; U. S. Bureau of Census, 1992). Most female farm operators are widowed or never married, putting them at risk for inadequate support in later years (Sachs, 1983).

Retirement Planning

Several factors explain the vulnerability of female farm operators to inadequate planning. Farm operators and self-employed workers in general are vulnerable to a lack of financial and social support in later life due to their limited access to retirement planning information (Kragie et al., 1989). Farmers also rely on professional help less than other workers (Martinez-Brawley & Blundall, 1989). Because of the patriarchal nature of the occupation, female farm operators rarely belong to the professional organizations providing farmers with even a minimal amount of assistance with retirement planning (Sachs, 1983).

When examining the social support planning of a specific occupational group such as farm women, several distinct variables may influence the degree to which they anticipate and plan for later life. This study examines the acceptability of informal social support options if health should fail in later years among aging women farm operators. It further examines the characteristics of the women farmers related to increased acceptability of a variety of informal social support options. By identifying which informal social support options farm women view as acceptable in later life, professionals and educators can more adequately prepare to offer assistance in the overall retirement planning process.

METHOD

The data for this project are part of a larger study examining retirement planning of farm operators over the age of 40 years living in Arkansas, Louisiana, Missouri, Mississippi, and Tennessee. The United States Department of Agriculture (USDA) Statistical Service in Little Rock, Arkansas collected the data through the Computer Assisted Telephone Interview (CATI) system. The population frame was from the USDA data base of individuals from the five states who reported gross farm sales of $20,000 or more in 1992. The sample selection process incorporated a multi-stage stratified random sampling procedure to select potential sample members.

A member of the USDA staff completed a telephone survey with the individual named in the USDA data base as the farm operator, thus assuring that the interviewed person legally was the farm operator. The interviewers asked all operators screening questions, to ensure that they were full-time farmers. Because the operators had frequent contact with the USDA statistical service and a high level of interest in the topics covered, the refusal rate of those who qualified to participate in the study was less than 10%. Sampling and screening procedures resulted in a total sample of 2,021 male and female farm operators. The data used in the present study came from the interviews with the 151 female farm operators.

Measure

The author developed a structured questionnaire for use in this study. The questionnaire assessed the acceptability of several social support options as well as health and demographic characteristics of the female farm operators.

Demographic Variables. The demographic variables examined were age, race, marital status, education level, and income. The interviewers also asked the respondents, "How many children under the age of 18 are living in the household?"

Informal Social Support. Seven questions assessed the acceptability of informal social support options in later life. These questions fell into two categories: in-home options and live-in options. The operators responded to the following, "In later years, help may be needed if health declines. There are many choices that we can have for our housing and the needed help and care. How acceptable would each of the following be to you?" They selected their response from among four response options: (0) not acceptable, (1) somewhat acceptable, (2) very acceptable, and (3) does not apply. For the analysis, "does not apply" equaled a missing response. The options for in-home support included having children or relatives come by to help, depending on spouse for help, and having a neighbor or friend come by to help. The options for informal live-in support in later life were: having relative(s) move in, moving to a mobile home or small home next to a child or relative, moving into the home of a child, and moving into the home of another relative. From these items, the author developed two additional measures. The in-home scale ranged from zero (all three options were unacceptable) to 6 (all three items were very acceptable). The live-in scale ranged from zero (all four choices were unacceptable) to eight (all four choices were very acceptable).

Health Status, Life Satisfaction, and Retirement Attitude. The interviewers asked the women to describe their perception of their current health. Possible responses were: poor, fair, good, or excellent. One global question assessed life satisfaction among the sample participants. Respondents were asked, "Right now, how do you feel about your life as a whole . . . On a 1 to 4 scale, with 1 being very dissatisfied and 4 being very satisfied, where would you fall?" Response options were: (1) very dissatisfied, (2) dissatisfied, (3) satisfied, and (4) very satisfied. Another global question ascertained respondents' attitude toward retirement. The interviewers asked the operators, "How do you feel about retirement from the farm?" Possible responses were: (1) Feel positive about retirement, (2) Feel somewhat neutral about retirement, (3) Feel negative about retirement, or (4) Don't know. "Don't know" was coded as missing for the purposes of analysis.

RESULTS

Sample Characteristics

The majority of the farm women were married (69.5%) and white (95.4%). The mean age was 59.9 years. Almost one-half of the women (44.4%) were high school graduates. Over one-third of the women (35.8%) reported a family income of over $80,000 in 1992; 39.8% reported incomes below $30,000. Over 83% of the sample reported having no children living at home at the time of the study. Most of the women (51.7%) reported that they were in "good" health. Most operators reported being satisfied (53.7%) or very satisfied (39.1%) with their current life as a whole. Table 1 presents further details of the demographic characteristics of the farm women.

The majority of the farm women (76.2%) said that being raised on a farm was "important" or "very important" in their decision to become a farm operator. Over 80% of the women had inherited their farm. However, 42% indicated that having a family farm available was not an important factor in their decision to farm. Most of the women (91%) lived on their farms, two-thirds of which were within 10 miles of town. The women had been on their farms for an average of 29 years and 80% of them said that they were unlikely to move from the farm in their later years. Fifty-three percent of the women had family members helping on the farm. However, only 49% expected to turn the farm over to a child at some time in the future.

Informal Social Support

Table 2 presents the level of acceptability of each of the informal help options. Of the in-home support options, depending on a spouse for help was the most acceptable form of social support with 86.5% of the married respondents saying spousal help was "very acceptable." The least acceptable in-home option was having a friend or neighbor come by to help, with 15% reporting that this was not an acceptable option and another 44.9% indicating that it was only "somewhat acceptable." The least acceptable live-in options were moving to the home of a child, with 76.9% reporting this as an unacceptable option, and moving to the home of another relative; 78.9% indicated this option was not acceptable. Although none of the live-in options were very acceptable to the farm women, the most acceptable option was having a relative move into the home. Almost 9% said this option was "very acceptable," and another 45.6% found it to be "somewhat acceptable."

ANOVAs were used to determine the acceptability of informal social support options as a result of several demographic characteristics: marital status, number of children under age 18 currently in the home, current health status, overall life satisfaction, age of the respondent, and total family living income. Tukey multiple range comparison tests were used to examine significant differences between groups.

In-Home Help. Respondents in poor health (n = 4) reported in-home support from a child as a "very acceptable" option. The women in good (n = 76) or excellent (n = 30) health viewed having a child come by to help to be a "somewhat" to "very acceptable" option ($F(3,142) = 2.69$, $p <$ .05). None of the other demographic characteristics differentiated between any of the informal in-home support options.

TABLE 1. Demographic Characteristics of the Sample

Variable	Frequency	Valid Percent
Age (*M* = 59.9)		
40-49	28	18.5%
50-59	43	28.5%
60-69	49	32.5%
70+	31	20.5%
Race		
White	144	95.4%
Black	7	4.6%
Marital Status		
Married	105	69.5%
Separated/Divorced	5	3.3%
Widowed	35	23.2%
Never Married	6	4.0%
Education Level		
8th Grade Or Less	10	6.9%
Less Than High School	23	16.0%
High School/GED	64	44.4%
Junior College/Technical School	6	4.2%
Some College	19	13.2%
Bachelors Degree	14	9.7%
Post-graduate Degree	8	5.6%
Income		
0-$14,999	17	11.3%
$15,000-29,999	43	28.5%
$30,000-49,999	26	17.2%
$50,000-79,999	11	7.3%
$80,000+	54	35.8%
Current Health Status		
Poor	4	2.6%
Fair	37	24.5%
Good	78	51.7%
Excellent	32	21.2%

TABLE 1 (continued)

Variable	Frequency	Valid Percent
Life as a Whole		
Very Dissatisfied	3	2.0%
Dissatisfied	8	5.3%
Satisfied	81	53.6%
Very Satisfied	59	39.1%
Number of Children Under Age 18 Living in the Household		
None	126	83.4%
One	11	7.3%
Two	10	6.6%
Three	3	2.0%
Four	1	0.7%
Plan to Retire from Farm		
Yes	61	40.4%
No	72	47.7%
Don't know	18	11.9%
Plan to Turn the Farm Over to Child		
Yes	74	49.0%
No	58	38.4%
Don't know	19	14.6%

Live-In Options. Although neither group found it very acceptable, married women found having a non-relative move in more acceptable than did the non-married women ($F(1,148) = 3.80$, $p < .05$). The total number of children under the age of 18 years still living in the home differentiated between the reported levels of acceptability for the option of moving into the home of a child ($F(4,138) = 2.68$, $p < .05$). Although the ANOVA was significant, the follow-up analysis showed that no two groups differed significantly.

Factors Related to Acceptability of Support Options. Over 80% of the women found three or more of the in-home options at least somewhat acceptable. Each of these scales was used as a dependent variable in a linear multiple regression analysis to determine which demographic factors were most predictive of overall higher levels of acceptability of in-home and live-in social support options. The independent variables were

TABLE 2. Acceptability of In-Home and Live-In Informal Help Options

Informal Options	Not Acceptable		Somewhat Acceptable		Very Acceptable	
In-home Options	N	%	N	%	N	%
Child help	11	7.5%	56	38.4%	79	54.1%
Spouse help (Married only)	7	6.7%	7	6.7%	90	86.5%
Neighbor/friend help	22	15.0%	66	44.9%	59	40.1%
Live-in Options						
Relative move in	67	45.6%	67	45.6%	13	8.8%
Non-relative move in	92	61.3%	52	34.7%	6	4.0%
Move near child or relative	76	52.8%	57	39.6%	11	7.6%
Move in with child	110	76.9%	29	20.3%	4	2.8%
Move to home of relative	116	78.9%	28	19.0%	3	2.0%

selected based on previous research in which these particular variables influenced retirement planning activities (Trenary, 1995; Turner, Bailey, & Scott, 1994). The independent variables in the analyses included overall life satisfaction, education level completed, attitudes toward retirement, race, income, number of children under the age of 18 remaining in the household, age of the respondent, and respondent's current self-perceived health status.

Because an in-home option on the scale was "depending on spouse for help," the in-home regression analysis included only the 104 married respondents in the study. The regression analysis examining the factors related to higher levels of acceptability of in-home sources of support was not significant ($F(8,86) = .96, p > .05$). Similarly, the regression analysis, exploring factors predictive of increased acceptability of the live-in support options, was not significant ($F(9,125) = .97, p > .05$). Neither of the regression analyses significantly explained differences in the acceptability of either in-home or live-in support options.

DISCUSSION

The purpose of this study was to examine a group of nontraditional aging women and their attitudes about the acceptability of specific social support options in later years. Further, the study sought to determine the personal factors related to levels of acceptability of specific in-home and live-in social support systems. Although more information is now available describing female farm operators, the results of the analysis examining factors differentiating the women in their acceptance of specific social support options are disappointing. Few of the demographic and attitude characteristics examined provided significant indications of factors differentiating between the women. However, some important conclusions can be drawn from the results of the study.

The women of this study are in non-traditional roles as women farm operators. Their high level of independence, which allows them to be successful in this role, can be seen in their intentions for their remaining years. The majority intend to stay on their farms, which may be as far from the nearest town as 45 miles. Their resistance to accept any help except from a spouse emphasizes their desire to remain independent. Their rejection of any of the live-in support options also reflects their strong desire to live independently for the remaining years of their lives. Although this resistance to in-home help or live-in support is not unique to this group of women but is rather common to many older adults, more of these female farm operators reported a lack of acceptance of any of the informal support options than university employees in a similar study (Turner, Roberto, & Bailey, 1988).

The findings do support previous research that indicates that people depend on their families for help more often than other sources (Scott & Roberto, 1985). Although the expectation is that friends and neighbors are strong sources of support in rural communities, having neighbors or friends provide assistance was the least acceptable in-home support. Over 60% of the women rejected the possibility of having a non-relative move into their home if they needed help. The women viewed spouses and then children as the most acceptable sources of support for in-home help, thus supporting the premise of the substitution model (Shanas, 1979). The high number of respondents (52.3%) indicating that moving next to a child was not an acceptable option is contrary to the myth of farm life that generations care for one another by sharing the land and living close to aging family members to provide any needed support. Perhaps this group of female farm operators has experienced caring for a parent or parent-in-law living nearby and thus chose to reject that as a means of support for themselves. Further, the mobility of farm children and the lack of availability of a child to take over the farm emphasizes the changing roles on the family farm.

The lack of significant findings related to levels of social support suggests that this is a very homogeneous group of women. Despite differences in marital status, income, education level, and other demographic characteristics, the attitudes and expectations of the women for the friend and family support systems in later life are remarkably similar. The factors that differentiate between the levels of acceptability of the various informal social support options are very likely qualitative rather than the quantitative factors assessed in this study. Previous life experiences on the farm and the quality of current family and friend relationships will more likely determine acceptable support options as these women age than the demographic and attitude characteristics they expressed in this study.

For these female farm operators, the blending of their work and family roles strongly influences their decisions for social support in later years. However, the findings of this study suggest the need for concern about the adequacy of the preparations these women are making for their social support needs in later years. The myth of life on the family farm clearly does not apply to many of these female farm operators.

IMPLICATIONS FOR FUTURE RESEARCH AND PRACTICE

The findings of this study suggest the need for further research related to the growing number of female farm operators and their preparations for the later years. The uniqueness of this group of nontraditional women requires an in-depth examination to discern their expectations and needs for their later years. Research needs to examine the qualitative issues related to the women's expectations for social support in later life. Interviews examining what life and relationships on the farm have meant and how those experiences have directed their future plans will provide essential insights. A longitudinal study following a group of women farm operators across the years as health and family concerns force them to make decisions regarding continuing as full-time farmers would greatly enrich the available literature.

Although 50% of all female farm operators live in the South, this study is limited in its ability to examine women from other geographic locations and different types and sizes of farms. Expanding the study to include women operating a variety of types of farms in different parts of the country would broaden the generalizability of the study. As the number of female farm operators continues to grow, further research will be essential to understand and respond to the needs of these women.

The practice implications of this study are diverse. Cooperative Extension agents, counselors, educators, and others who assist these farm operators with their retirement plans need to be aware of the importance of social support in later years. They need to develop programs designed to fit the individual needs of the female farmer approaching retirement. Female farm operators must assess their current relationships. Further, they must realize that their plans for independent living on the farm for the rest of their lives may not be possible because of unexpected health problems requiring some assistance. They must take responsibility for planning for necessary support to maintain the independence and quality of life that is so important to them. Identifying and planning for all aspects of the retirement process will enable female farm operators to make the transition into later life more successfully.

REFERENCES

Antonucci, T. C., & Akiyama, H. (1987). An examination of sex differences in social support among older men and women. *Sex Roles, 17,* 737-749.

Bailey, W. C., & Turner, M. J. (1994). Significance of sources of retirement planning information for farmers. *Financial Counseling and Planning, 5,* 83-99.

Cantor, M. H. (1983). Strain among caregivers: A study of experience in the United States. *The Gerontologist, 23,* 597-611.

Dwyer, J. W., Lee, G. R., & Coward, R. T. (1990). The health status, health services utilization, and support networks of the rural elderly: A decade review. *The Journal of Rural Health, 6,* 379-398.

Gallagher, E., & Delworth, U. (1993). The third shift: Juggling employment, family, and the farm. *Journal of Rural Community Psychology, 12*(2), 21-38.

Gasson, R., & Winter, M. (1992). Gender relations and farm household pluractivity. *Journal of Rural Studies, 8,* 387-397.

Geisler, C. C., Waters, W. F., & Eadie, K. L. (1985). The changing structure of female agricultural land ownership, 1946-1978. *Rural Sociology, 50*(1), 74-87.

Kalbacher, J. Z. (1983). Women farm operators. *Family Economics Review, 4,* 17-21.

Kalbacher, J. Z. (1985). A profile of female farmers in America. *Rural Development Research Report,* No. 45. Washington, DC: United States Department of Agriculture.

Kivett, V. R. (1990). Older rural women: Mythical, forbearing, and unsung. *Journal of Rural Community Psychology, 11*(1), 83-101.

Kosberg, J. I., & Cairl, R. E. (1986). The cost of care index: A case management tool for screening informal care providers. *The Gerontologist, 26,* 273-278.

Kragie, E. R., Gerstein, M., & Lichtman, M. (1989). Do Americans plan for retirement? Some recent trends. *Career Development Quarterly, 37,* 232-239.

Kramer, J. S. (1991). *Who cares for the elderly?* New York: Garland Publishing.

Krause, N. (1990). Perceived health problems, formal/informal support, and life satisfaction among older adults. *Journals of Gerontology, 45,* S193-S205.

Leckie, G. J. (1993). Female farmers in Canada and the gender relations of a restructuring agricultural system. *The Canadian Geographer, 37,* 212-230.

Martinez-Brawley, E., & Blundall, J. (1989). Farm families' preferences toward the personal social services. *Social Work, 34,* 513-522.

Mercier, J. M., Paulson, L., & Morris, E. W. (1988). Rural and urban elderly: Differences in the quality of the parent-child relationship. *Family Relations, 37,* 68-72.

Peters, G. R., Hoyt, D. R., Babchuk, N., Kaiser, M., & Iijima, Y. (1987). Primary-group support systems of the aged. *Research on Aging, 9,* 392-416.

Pilisuk, M., & Parks, S. H. (1988). Caregiving: Where families need help. *Social Work, 33,* 436-440.

Rosenfeld, R. A. (1985). *Farm women. Work, farm, and family in the United States.* Chapel Hill: University of North Carolina Press.

Sachs, C. E. (1983). *The invisible farmers: Women in agricultural production.* Totowa, NJ: Rowman & Allanheld.

Scott, J. P., & Roberto, K. A. (1985). Use of informal and formal support networks by rural elderly poor. *The Gerontologist, 25,* 624-630.

Shanas, E. (1979). The family as a social support system in old age. *The Gerontologist, 19,* 169-174.

Stoller, E. P., & Pugliesi, K. L. (1988). Informal networks of community-based elderly. *Research on Aging, 10,* 499-516.

Trenary, L. A. (1995). *Retirement planning among midlife farm operators.* Unpublished master's thesis, University of Arkansas, Fayetteville, Arkansas.

Turner, M. J. (1993). Retirement planning behaviors among Arkansas farm families. *Arkansas Farm Research Journal, 42*(3), 8-9.

Turner, M. J., Bailey, W. C., & Scott, J. P. (1994). Factors influencing attitude toward retirement and retirement planning among midlife university employees. *Journal of Applied Gerontology, 13,* 143-156.

Turner, M. J., Roberto, K. A., & Bailey, W. C. (1988, September). Midlife planning for the use of social supports in late life. Paper presented at Fifth National Forum on Research in Aging, Lincoln, NE.

U.S. Bureau of the Census. (1992). *Census of Agriculture, 1, Geographic Area Series, Part 51.* Washington, DC: U.S. Department of Commerce, Economic & Statistics Administration.

U.S. Bureau of the Census. (1993). *Statistical Abstract of the United States: 1993* (113th ed.). Washington, DC: Author

Empowerment-Oriented Social Work Practice: Impact on Late Life Relationships of Women

Enid Opal Cox, DSW
Ruth R. Parsons, PhD

SUMMARY. Empowerment interventions promote egalitarian, strengths-based relationships through education, self-help, mutual support, consciousness raising, and social action activities. In this paper we describe the influence of empowerment-oriented group intervention on the relationships of older women. We conducted qualitative interviews with the women who participated in the group and the social workers who staffed the intervention activities. The findings suggest that, in addition to other empowerment outcomes, the older women participants developed sustaining relationships with each other and often seriously considered the nature of their other late life relationships. Thus, empowerment-oriented interventions can enhance the quality of life for older women, including the development and support of meaningful interpersonal relationships. *[Article copies available from The Haworth Document Delivery Service: 1-800-342-9678. E-mail address: getinfo@haworth.com]*

Enid Opal Cox is Professor and Director, Institute of Gerontology, Graduate School of Social Work, and Ruth R. Parsons is Professor, Graduate School of Social Work, both at the University of Denver, Denver, CO 80208.

[Haworth co-indexing entry note]: "Empowerment-Oriented Social Work Practice: Impact on Late Life Relationships of Women." Cox, Enid Opal and Ruth R. Parsons. Co-published simultaneously in the *Journal of Women & Aging* (The Haworth Press, Inc.) Vol. 8, Nos. 3/4, 1996, pp. 129-143; and: *Relationships Between Women in Later Life* (ed: Karen A. Roberto) The Haworth Press, Inc., 1996, pp. 129-143; and: *Relationships Between Women in Later Life* (ed: Karen A. Roberto) Harrington Park Press, an imprint of The Haworth Press, Inc., 1996, pp. 129-143. [Single or multiple copies of this article are available from the Haworth Document Delivery Service: 1-800-342-9678, 9:00 a.m. - 5:00 p.m. (EST). E-mail address: getinfo@haworth.com]

In this paper we describe empowerment-oriented social work practice and the relationship of this practice model to late life relationships among older women who participate in empowerment-oriented programs. Three key aspects of empowerment-oriented practice relate strongly to the nature of late life relationships: (a) the philosophy and goals of empowerment-oriented practice, (b) the use of small groups as a preferred modality for empowerment-oriented interventions, and (c) the nature of interpersonal relationships supported by empowerment-oriented practice strategies.

Empowerment philosophy has emphasized the importance of collaborative problem definition and decision-making, collective action, client strengths, education, mutual aid and self-help activities, and resource access. Personal problems and challenges are social constructs related to one's political environment. Values promoted by empowerment-oriented philosophy include: a more egalitarian distribution of resources and power, more egalitarian relationships (including the reduction of racism, ageism, homophobia, discrimination based on disability, and other forms of discrimination), democratic processes, and concern for the ecological environment. Consequently, strategies to increase a sense of efficacy often require involvement (i.e., relationships) with others (Cox & Parsons, 1994; Dunst, Trivette, & LaPointe, 1992; Gutierrez, 1988, 1990).

Interpersonal relationships represent a bond (i.e., uniting force or agreement) in which both individuals acknowledge a connection between them. Such a relationship requires continued interaction to develop and contains the following basic substantive components or dimensions (Miller, 1986): (a) Belonging and affirmation–approval, acceptance, a sense of membership, value consensus, responsibility, companionship; (b) Interdependence/aid–exchange of resources, goods, finances, knowledge, time and effort; and (c) Intimacy/affect–mutual attraction and liking, trust, love, respect, enabling, and shared confidence.

The framework necessary for individuals to engage in empowering experiences depends upon the creation of relationships containing these components and participation in the activities. We describe these activities in our discussion of empowerment-oriented groups.

Empowerment is a process through which individuals and groups become strong enough to participate within, share in the control of, and influence events and institutions affecting their lives. It also is a process through which individuals gain more control of and/or the ability to make positive changes in the personal, interpersonal and/or political aspects of their lives (Cox & Parsons, 1994; Torre, 1985). The empowerment process contains three key components (Cox & Parsons, 1994; Kieffer, 1981, 1984):

1. The critical examination of attitudes, values and beliefs, including those related to self-efficacy, self-esteem, self-worth, and belief in self as well as one's understanding of the interpersonal and political aspects of their problems/issues.
2. The development of knowledge, skills and networking with others toward mutual support, education and problem solving.
3. Taking action on behalf of oneself and others, based on a critical and collective perspective of one's issues.

Empowerment interventions with elders have received increasing attention in the last decade (Akins, 1985; Cohen, 1990; Cox, 1988; Cox & Parsons, 1994; Maze, 1987). Empowerment interventions have emphasized both the curative and preventive aspects of empowerment. Most views of empowerment-oriented practice stress the advantages of the use of small groups as the most effective modality of practice for the promotion of empowerment. The opportunity to participate in small empowerment-oriented groups also has an important impact on interpersonal relationships of the group members.

EMPOWERMENT-ORIENTED SMALL GROUPS AND INTERPERSONAL RELATIONSHIPS

Small groups are a modality that greatly enhances efforts to engage clients in empowerment activity (Cox & Parsons, 1994; Gutierrez, 1990). Goals of empowerment-oriented groups include: (a) the development of mutual support and self-help among members; (b) education, including knowledge and skills, for survival and coping with life's challenges; (c) development of skills of critical analysis and a critical perspective on one's life struggles within their environmental context; and (d) collective social action. Activities geared toward these goals often occur simultaneously, depending on the process and activities of the group, but always in the context of on-going consciousness raising/problem assessment by the group. Pernell (1986) summarized these points well when she said:

> Groups are a natural context for efforts toward empowerment. They are a collective with the resources of several people and of program content; contributions made to the whole and received from the whole. The group can be an opportunity system with its inner resources and its collective strength for acquisition of external resources. (p. 114)

Empowerment-based small group interventions with older women (Cox & Parsons, 1994) have stressed the importance of interpersonal relationships and the importance of a cohesive collective or group experience to problem solving. Browne (1992) reminds us that older women have different affiliative needs than older men. Specifically, older women place more emphasis on connection and relationship, collective and community good, in recognition and response to their social power reality of inequality. She suggests that empowerment of older women means a reframing of power from its traditional conceptualization in aging as control and independence as markers of successful aging (Rodenheaver, 1987 as cited in Browne, 1992). Browne further recommends that newer conceptions of power must include social support, friendship, community connections, self-help, collective action and increased ability to engage in critical thinking. This perspective focuses on the development of knowledge and skills for interdependent relationships. It emphasizes coping by developing new relationships and restructuring old ones to involve mutuality and reciprocity. Most empowerment-oriented groups focused on issues of older adults include specific curriculum devoted to the discussion of social support in late life, including the importance of social support and ways to develop and sustain support networks.

Another value of empowerment-oriented practice important to participation in empowerment groups is the egalitarian nature of relationships. Group leaders seek to develop an egalitarian relationship with their group members and to foster egalitarian relationships among members as they participate in interventions. The emphasis is on egalitarian relationships in caregiving/care-receiving interactions, and among group members engaged in mutual action.

In the following section we describe a typical empowerment-oriented care-receiver intervention project and report the findings of a post-hoc study of the perceptions of the elderly women participants. Their perceptions of their experiences provide several examples of the impact of this participation on their interpersonal relationships. The process and findings of this study are described and analyzed in terms of this impact.

THE INTERVENTION

We initiated a small group empowerment intervention project in a Catholic operated low-income housing complex in 1992. This complex includes two free standing senior independent living facilities and an assisted living facility. A Master's level social worker, with empowerment and gerontology training and experience, implemented the intervention under the supervision of a social work professor and the senior program director for the facility. The goals of this project were to: (a) engage semi-isolated elders in a process that enhanced their understanding and knowledge concerning increased dependence due to loss and the normative aging process; (b) identify and increase coping skills related to this challenge; and (c) facilitate older adults' participation in mutual aid, social action and other meaningful activities that promote the empowerment process.

The intervention program consisted of a small group empowerment process. Approximately ten elderly women and two elderly men participated in the initial phase of the project. Most members of the group were over 75 years old. All members experienced one or more of the common physical conditions of aging (e.g., arthritis, loss of hearing or sight, heart problems and frailty). One elder was legally blind and two used walkers.

Participants were residents of three different facilities (buildings). The group meetings occurred bi-monthly. Group activities included consciousness raising, socialization, self-help, education, and social action. The group members decided the content of the meetings. The group leader shared ideas regarding content generated from similar groups (e.g., health care issues, professional/client communications issues and strategies). The issues addressed by the group emerged as the group members began to interact and discuss issues of concern to them. Issues that the group pursued over time included information about Medicare, Medicaid, local clinics, experiences with doctors and other health professionals, how to get information from health professionals, and communications with children. The group members also engaged in self-help processes such as searching and comparing prices for drugs, finding transportation resources, and accompanying each other to doctors' offices to assure clear communications. They also engaged in discussions about their roots, family history, early childhood experiences, the use of humor and other strategies for coping with late life challenges (e.g., increased dependency). At times the members also discussed political aspects of senior resources or their children's and grandchildren's circumstances.

The University-based team sponsored the group for approximately seven months. At that point, the senior services coordinator for the facility and a younger group member (54 year-old woman with a disability) assumed responsibility for the intervention. Three years after initiation of the intervention, we conducted a post-hoc qualitative study to explore the empowerment experience of older female participants in this empowerment project. At the time of the post-hoc study, the group was still meeting monthly.

OLDER WOMEN'S PERSPECTIVE
OF THE EMPOWERMENT EXPERIENCE

We used qualitative methods to understand the processes involved in receiving help in an empowerment-based program, and to learn how older women described the effects of the program on themselves. We solicited unique responses and common or thematic responses from the women.

Sampling and Data Gathering

The second author (Parsons) obtained permission to attend a meeting of the empowerment group and to interview the eight members who attended that session together in a focus group format. The purpose of the group interview was to determine what the program was like, how the members had experienced it, and what they could identify as changes in themselves because of participating in the group. We used a general interview guide to direct the questions. After consultation with the staff and resident leaders, four older women participants were selected for individual, in-depth interviews. These participants demonstrated capacity to express themselves and articulate the experience; they also had longevity in the group.

The researcher and a Ph.D. student conducted the interviews. We used the general interview guide approach (Patton, 1987) to direct the questions. It included the history of the women, what led them to the program, what they had hoped to gain, what the experience had been like, how they experienced the program staff, and what factors in their experience had been most helpful and life changing. Participants received $10.00 for the interview. All interviews were audio-taped and transcribed.

Study Participants

The eight group members who participated in the focus group interview were all white women, ages 76 and over, except for one member/leader who was younger (age 58) and disabled. Their lengths of time in the group ranged from nine months to three years (i.e., since the beginning of the group). Four members of the focus group participated in the individual interview component of the study; three of the women were in their early 80's and one younger woman (age 58) was both a member and a resident leader in the group. These participants had been involved in the group since its beginning.

Analysis

We analyzed the transcripts from the group interview and the individual in-depth interviews together. Through repeated readings, we extracted ideas from the transcripts and organized them into categories. From these categories, we identified distinct themes and the relationship among themes (Patton, 1990). We use direct quotes from the women to support these themes.

RESULTS

Relationship Components

The following relationship components emerged from discussions with the older women: a safe environment, opportunity for interaction, commonality, interdependence, support and acceptance, expression of feelings, mutual education, mutual aid, role modeling, collective decision making and problem solving, and taking collective action. These themes reflect compatibility and confirmation of Miller's (1986) research mentioned earlier regarding the components of relationship.

Participants stressed the importance of *feeling safe* in the group. They described the group as an opportunity for interaction with others in a safe and supportive place. As one participant said, "It just feels good to go there and be with those other women; it is a safe place."

The *opportunity to interact* with others, or, as one participant phrased it, "the opportunity to reach outside yourself" was important to the development of a cohesive collective among the participants. The women viewed socialization and staying involved with others as important for happiness and keeping their social skills active. One woman said, "I just wanted to have an hour of pleasure in my day."

Interaction with each other seemed to help develop a sense of *commonality.* The women identified the feeling of being "all in the same boat," and the comfort of knowing that "you are not alone" as important aspects of group interaction. The following comments from the women support this theme:

It's helpful even to find out that others are struggling with the same issues . . . I thought it was all me.

I guess other people's children act the same way mine do . . . that helped me cope with it.

It is easier to talk about things with people who have the same issues. I found myself talking about things I never could before.

A sense of commonality seemed to create a supportive atmosphere and fostered the expression of feelings. The women referred to *support* as acceptance, being nurtured, having trust, being encouraged and being challenged. They also described support as appreciating what each one does for the other, giving hugs, discussion, getting advice, and knowing someone is listening when you need to talk. Elizabeth, age 84, and increasingly losing her eyesight said:

> Yes, I love to be with people. It is good for my morale. I can get cabin crazy, but every time we have that meeting, the rest of the day goes with ease. We just be kind, lovable, considerate to each other. People can express their views of life and we learn what each of us is dealing with and try to help each other.

Another woman, age 83, strong, and assertive, who was previously a buyer for a department store, commented:

> You learn to get along with people a little better by listening to all their frailties; you have a little more charity toward people. It helps you to hear other people's troubles . . . we have been meeting over a year and we have grown much closer . . . it is shared commitment— we are all trying to do some of the same things in our lives.

Expression of feelings is a major part of relationship building, and according to the women, it meant that they were heard and listened to. For example, one woman said, "I talked about things I never have before–you know, being afraid or angry." The women could reach inside and let their feelings out and receive support for those feelings. Norma, age 83, who had a successful career and whose husband had died in the last five years said:

> Talking about all you've lost and your grief helps you and relieves your stress. Everyone knows how you feel and they can understand because they are going through it also, then you don't feel so bad.

A supportive group creates an opportunity for interdependence. The women described *interdependence* as mutual dependence, assuming responsibility for the well-being of each other, collective support, mutual aid, and problem solving. It fosters a new level of responsibility in the women members.

Although society promotes independence, older women find that interdependence becomes more and more necessary in order not to simply be dependent. Discussion of interdependence with the women brought the following comments. Violet, an active volunteer, retired from a career in business and fashion, with severe loss of hearing said:

> The little lady that I read to–she also helps me. She said that I read to her and she hears for me. She repeats things for me so that I can hear them. I learned that there are other people who like to exchange also.

Elizabeth, who is losing her sight, commented:

> Sometimes you think I can't help nobody else. I can't even help myself, but then you see that listening and understanding other people's situation does help them and then you don't feel so bad about you know, leaning on others a little.

Studying and learning collectively was one of the most often mentioned benefits of the group as far as bringing about change. Education and skill development for coping with aging were key objectives of the project. Comments, such as the following from Norma who was dealing with loss of her husband and her own health issues, reflect these objectives:

> Well, we all talk about our frailties and aging and you get a lot out of that by listening to somebody else's . . . you learn to cope with your own a little bit . . . we call about good grocery prices, transportation resources, and all that gets brought back to the group. And, if you forget, you know who to ask to remind you. These people are like your family and when they die, it is like losing a family member, but I have learned from the group about losing your loved ones and how to cope with grief. Having people to come in and tell us about Medicare was so informative because it is so hard to understand.

Violet, who had always been a giver instead of a receiver said, "I have learned that people have tried all kinds of things that I never heard of."

Mutual decision-making was prominent in the women's descriptions of what occurred in their groups. One active volunteer stated:

> We have many committees made up of residents and staff who make decisions for the facility. Everyone needs to know about these things because it affects us all.

Another woman described it in this way:

> In our group, we decided what things we wanted to learn about–for example, we had someone come and talk to us about depression around Christmas time. We all learned some ideas about preventing depression. It was easy to agree on things we wanted to do or hear about because most of us had the same problems.

The women saw themselves as *role models* for each other as they described the importance of watching and learning from others who are or have been in the same boat. The women made the following observations:

> Some of the people here are nicer and kinder than I am and I try to learn a lot from them.

> There is something about the way she handles what life deals her that inspires me to be more patient and try harder.

> If you have any weakness in your character and you see another person that doesn't have that weakness, it makes you say "why can't I be like her." It gives you the desire to do better, to make something of yourself.

The women described *mutual problem solving* efforts by the group members. They spoke of finding solutions to problems, figuring out alternatives, making choices and acting on them. For example, one woman stated:

> The thing that helped me the most was the transportation problems. We discussed and suggested this and that and I found a lady to take me to the eye doctor and sit and wait for me, take me to the dentist and drag me in and out and the transportation was solved.

Another woman said:

> That is another thing we discussed, how to deal with maintenance problems. I had that drippy faucet and we got it fixed.

Elizabeth, concerned with medical problems, provided the following example:

> Well, it helped me when I go to the doctor. I don't know why I get so brainless, I forget what I am going to ask him . . . but, I try to think

two or three days before I go what it is that I want to ask him. We set up a system of going to the doctor together so two of us could slow him down and be sure we got all our questions answered.

Norma commented:

When one of us found out about a resource we shared it with the whole group. We help each other with problems in this group. We make tapes for . . . because she can't see . . . and we help each other cope with losses and grieve in a good way.

Accessing and connecting with resources is a necessary skill for older women. The empowerment group helped them with this need. One woman reported:

Call transportation is one thing I do better and the prescriptions . . . The Medicare thing can drive you to distraction. I've been frustrated to where I want to scream. This has helped me know a bit better what to do.

Mutual learning also meant learning from each other. Elizabeth commented:

It amazed me how much we knew when we put our heads together.

The women talked about gaining understanding of their problem(s) and where they came from and about educating and helping others. Limited by frail physical conditions and receiving assisted living services, these women expect themselves to *give back and make a contribution* instead of being the constant recipient. The staff facilitated this expectation as was evident in the comments of the women. For example, Norma said:

. . . and I try, because I get government aid, to do my part and watch the prices, and not be greedy, not just reach out and grab, but do my part to make it all work. I use as many generic drugs as I can; I have learned a lot about what I can do to help others.

Violet talked about her work in the facility:

We have fund-raisers and bake-sales and raise money. We give it to the Cancer Association, Heart Association, and the flood victims. You have to do what you are capable of doing, you know, to give

> back, when people are giving to you. I spend part of my day figuring
> out what can I do for somebody else.

Elizabeth added:

> Well, I can't do much, but I try to meet the new ones who come in
> and tell them my door is always open and I will be here when they
> need someone to talk to. Since I am blind, I can't do much, but I do
> what I can . . . I help this other blind lady on this floor. She is
> depressed about being blind and I reach out to her when I can.

The women described changed behavior and changes in knowledge and
beliefs. One behavioral change was *taking action* on their own behalf or
behalf of others. This included working for the general community and
joining organizations. One woman stated:

> I have been a delegate to the resident council for five years. We have
> a meeting once a month which we type up and let the others know
> what went on. We go over house rules, and problems and concerns.
> Everybody who lives here ought to know what is going on.

Another woman spoke about becoming more assertive in relation to her
health care:

> The druggist where my doctor is gave me a prescription, a name
> brand for $77.00. When I got home, I called another pharmacist who
> told me that the generic was $10.00. So, I got a refund and I got the
> generic. Now, I always tell my doctor to write the generic.

Politically active most of her life, Elizabeth described why she joined an
organization:

> I joined AARP because I like to have a voice in what goes on, maybe
> not a big one, but there are certain things you should be for and
> against and you need a place to be heard.

The themes suggest that women build relationships upon feelings of
trust, safety, and commonality. They developed through continued interaction and a sense of belonging, acceptance, affirmation, the capacity to
participate, interdependence, mutual aid, mutual decision making, and
mutual problem solving. A strong sense of wanting to contribute and give
back came from the relationship of reciprocity.

Group Leaders' Perspectives

We also interviewed the social worker who initiated and led the project during the first year and the program director of the housing project, who has served continuously as co-facilitator of the group, regarding their perceptions of the impact of the empowerment-oriented group participation on elderly group members. We asked them to address changes in the women's behaviors and beliefs. These included changes in relationships among group members or those reported by group members related to changes in relationships outside the group, but related to group activities. Their observations were as follows:

1. Individual women who had been somewhat isolated became increasingly active group participants.
2. Most women within the group established at least one close on-going friendship with other group member(s) over time.
3. Women who were quiet during first meetings became more involved when group topics related to areas of their competence and experience (positive response to strengths-based approach).
4. The egalitarian nature or value that guided group and worker interactions strengthened member-to-member respect and reinforced the strengths-based approach described above.
5. Sharing ideas about ways of coping with late life challenges reinforced these mutual support and egalitarian behaviors.
6. The group focus on self-help or helping others was helpful in motivating some women to become involved.
7. The identification of problems/issues as "common" problems appeared to help some women who tended to blame themselves to focus on problem solving instead of self-blame.
8. Participation in educational activities that emphasized the knowledge and experience (strengths) of group members as well as outside resources (e.g., learning about medical and financial resources and skills for communicating with medical professionals) appeared to stimulate participation and a sense of confidence that they could replicate successful experiences they heard about in the group.
9. Self-help activity such as going with each other to doctors or finding and sharing resources (transportation or responsive senior clinics) tended to promote a sense of hope and respect among the women.
10. Activities and information that occurred in the group setting began to affect other residents who were not group members. For example, they shared resources with friends and acquaintances not in the

group, and the women reported engaging in helping activities with others.

CONCLUSIONS AND IMPLICATIONS FOR PRACTICE AND RESEARCH

Empowerment-oriented practice developed based on the principles of egalitarian client-worker relationships, strengths-based assessment, the promotion of empowerment through education and skills development, consciousness-raising, self-help, and the use of collective and social action. Elderly participants in empowerment-oriented groups are encouraged to share concerns and issues that lead to a sense of "common problems/issues." Sharing one's problem with others often serves as a powerful stimulant with respect to diminishing self-blame for circumstances often beyond the control of elder group members. Participants share problem solution strategies with one another and promote a respect for individual strengths. The impact of this process on late life relationships is often two-fold. First, elderly group members are often more likely to share problems when they understand the environmental political aspects of their situation. Second, energy directed toward self-blame or the perception that one should "hide" problems becomes released and used for problem-solving activities. In empowerment-oriented groups, this energy often goes into the establishment of stronger interpersonal relationships and mutual aid activities. The sharing of strategies for solutions often leads to successful coping, skill development and a greater sense of competence among group members. These activities also have a positive influence on the establishment of late life relationships by promoting a sense of reciprocity and mutual respect.

The experience of elderly women who participate in empowerment-oriented interventions appears to support research that has emphasized the importance of social support and psychosocial factors in general health and mental health late in life. Group activity visibly leads to health education, increased social support, pro-active attention to depression, and other activities that promote health and mental health practice with older adults. The emphasis of these interventions on client strengths, development of knowledge and skills, critical assessment of issues and social action holds great promise for increased competency of elders who participate in these groups. Specific implications for practice include: (a) the use of small groups is a very viable strategy for work with frail older women; (b) ongoing participatory strengths-based problem assessment and participation in self-help, mutual-help activities promotes competence in coping with late life challenges; and (c) empowerment-oriented interventions can enhance the quality of life for older women including the development and support of meaningful interpersonal relationships. Because only a few pilot demonstrations of empowerment-oriented interventions have been recorded there is a great need for more practice-based research related to empowerment-oriented interventions. These intervention research efforts must clearly describe the process and outcomes of the projects they evaluate.

REFERENCES

Akins, T. E. (1985). Empowerment: Fostering independence of the older adult. *Aging Network News, 2*(5), 1-10.

Browne, C. (1992). *Empowerment in social work practice with older women.* Unpublished manuscript.

Cohen, E. S. (1990). The elderly mystique: Impediment to advocacy and empowerment. *Generations, 14,* (Supplement), 13-16.

Cox, E. O. (1988). Empowerment of the low income elderly through group work. *Social Work with Groups, 11*(3/4), 111-125.

Cox, E. O., & Parsons, R. J. (1994). *Empowerment oriented social work practice with the elderly.* Pacific Grove, CA: Brooks/Cole.

Dunst, C., Trivette, C. M., & LaPointe, N. (1992). Toward clarification of the meaning and key elements of empowerment. *Family Science Review, 5*(1/2), 111-130.

Gutierrez, L. M. (1988). *Empowerment in social work practice: Considerations for practice and education.* Paper presented to the Council on Social Work Education's Annual Program Meeting, Chicago, IL.

Gutierrez, L. M. (1990). Working with women of color: An empowerment perspective. *Social Work, 35*(2), 149-154.

Kieffer, P. C. (1981). *The emergence of empowerment: The development of participatory competence among individuals in citizen organizations.* Unpublished doctoral dissertation, University of Michigan, Ann Arbor.

Kieffer, P. C. (1984). Citizen empowerment: A developmental perspective. *Prevention in Human Services, 3,* 9.

Maze, T. (1987). Empowerment: Reflections on theory and practice. *Aging Network News, 4*(5).

Miller, S. (1986). Conceptualizing interpersonal relationships. *Generations, 10*(4), 6-9.

Patton, M. Q. (1987). *How to use qualitative methods in evaluation* (2nd ed.). Newbury Park, CA: Sage.

Patton, M. Q. (1990). *Qualitative evaluation and research methods* (2nd ed.), Newbury Park, CA: Sage.

Pernell, R. (1986). *Innovations in social group work: Feedback from practice to theory.* New York: Hanover.

Torre, D. (1985). *Empowerment: Structured conceptualization and instrument development.* Unpublished doctoral dissertation, Cornell University, New York.

The Guardianship Experience of Women: The Relationship Between Older Wards and Their Guardians

Robbyn R. Wacker, PhD
Pat M. Keith, PhD

SUMMARY. This research examined how 156 female legal caregivers responded to difficulties of being a guardian, how they derived meaning from their guardianship activities, and how the role of guardian influenced their perception of aging. The most frequent activities in which guardians engaged were visiting, providing emotional support, and to a lesser extent, giving instrumental assistance. Guardians described their emotional relationships with their wards as either "sympathetic," "sad," "challenged," or "hostile." Despite hardships associated with the duties of being a guardian, most of the women perceived benefits and expressed satisfaction from this role. Guardians reported that the relationship with their female wards shaped their perception of aging and the conception of their own aging. *[Article copies available from The Haworth Document Delivery Service: 1-800-342-9678. E-mail address: getinfo@haworth.com]*

Guardianships are sought when it is determined that an individual, commonly referred to as the "ward," is no longer competent to make

Robbyn R. Wacker is Associate Professor of Gerontology and Assistant Dean of the College of Health and Human Sciences, University of Northern Colorado, Greeley, CO 80639.

Pat M. Keith is Professor of Sociology and Assistant Dean of the Graduate College, Iowa State University, Ames, IA 50011.

[Haworth co-indexing entry note]: "The Guardianship Experience of Women: The Relationship Between Older Wards and Their Guardians." Wacker, Robbyn R. and Pat M. Keith. Co-published simultaneously in the *Journal of Women & Aging* (The Haworth Press, Inc.) Vol. 8, Nos. 3/4, 1996, pp. 145-158; and: *Relationships Between Women in Later Life* (ed: Karen A. Roberto) The Haworth Press, Inc., 1996, pp. 145-158; and: *Relationships Between Women in Later Life* (ed: Karen A. Roberto) Harrington Park Press, an imprint of The Haworth Press, Inc., 1996, pp. 145-158. [Single or multiple copies of this article are available from the Haworth Document Delivery Service: 1-800-342-9678, 9:00 a.m. - 5:00 p.m. (EST). E-mail address: getinfo@haworth.com] responsible decisions about his or her own welfare. A person obtains guardianship by filing a petition with the court of proper jurisdiction. At the hearing, evidence of the need for a guardian must be presented; the court must then make a determination for the need and scope of the guardianship. Many writers have voiced concerns in the legal and academic literature about the guardianship process, the inappropriate use of guardianship and the lack of court supervision of guardians (Bulcroft, Kielkopf, & Tripp, 1991; Hommel, Wang, & Bergman, 1990; Keith & Wacker, 1994). There has been little attention paid, however, to the experiences of guardians.

Researchers have documented that caregiving is primarily a woman's endeavor. Wives, daughters and daughters-in-law provide the majority of instrumental and emotional support to their elderly relatives (Stone, Cafferata, & Sangl, 1987). Sisters and other female relatives often are caregivers as well. In addition, many of these women find themselves with a formal caregiving duty–that of being a legal guardian. Furthermore, researchers indicate that caregiving affects the caregiver both personally and emotionally. For example, caregiving influences their relationship with their care receivers and other family members and the amount of burden and stress they experience (Walker, Martin, & Jones, 1992). We focus our investigation on the experiences of women who have the legal responsibility of caring for elderly women.

GUARDIANSHIP AS CAREGIVING

An extensive amount of research exists that examines the influence of caring on the lives of those who care for the aged (Dwyer & Coward, 1992; Pearlin, Mullan, Semple, & Skaff, 1990; Walker, Martin, & Jones, 1992). Caregivers provide emotional and instrumental support to the older adults they care for, with most caregivers providing care seven days per week (Stone, Cafferata, & Sangl, 1987). As a result, stress, role overload, and altered relationships have been especially salient concerns to researchers. Outcomes of caregiving include considerable financial, emotional and economic strain (Clipp & George, 1990; Scharlach & Boyd, 1989; Zarit, Todd, & Zarit, 1986). Besides the instrumental tasks performed by guardians, research on caregiving suggests that caregivers derive meaning from their duties (Hasselkus, 1988). For example, in an ethnographic study of caregivers, Hasselkus (1988) described five meanings of caregiving: sense of self, sense of managing, sense of fear and risk, sense of change in role and responsibility, and sense of future.

Although there are similarities between the activities and experiences of guardians and caregivers who are not legal guardians, there are also differences that might result in a unique type of caregiving experience for guardians. Guardianship, as legalized caregiving, entails a formalized relationship with the court that requires oversight of caregiving activities, and often the submission of reports detailing activities conducted on behalf of the ward. Besides having family members who may scrutinize caregiving activities, guardians now have additional scrutiny of their activities by the court. Furthermore, with the determination of incapacity of the ward, guardians make public the physical and/or mental decline of their family member. Obtaining guardianship also serves to recognize the role reversal of caregiver and care receiver, especially if the ward and guardian are parent and child. Thus, certain unique aspects of the guardianship role likely will generate strain particular to guardians, while the caregiving demands of guardians and the meaning caregivers derive from their activities may be similar to those experienced by other caregivers.

Although the literature provides documentation of the activities and outcomes of informal family caregiving, we know little about the experience of family and friends who provide legal caregiving. Therefore, the purpose of this paper is to examine this specific caregiving relationship. The following questions guided our investigation: (a) What activities do guardians engage in for their wards? (b) How do these women, as legal caregivers, respond to difficulties of being a guardian? (c) How and in what way do these women derive meaning from their guardianship activities? (d) What benefits and hardships do persons experience when fulfilling this legal caregiving role? and (e) How does the role of guardian influence these women's perception of aging?

METHOD

Sample

The data used in this study were collected as a part of a larger study about guardianship in Colorado, Iowa and Missouri (Keith & Wacker, 1994). We examined the court records of guardianships involving wards 60 years of age and older. Information garnered from the court records included the name and address of the guardian and information about guardian activities conducted for the ward. Since court records contained only cursory information about the guardians themselves, we sent all guardians a questionnaire that asked for more specific information as to the full extent of their activities and perceptions. Forty-nine percent (387) of the guardians returned their questionnaire. For this study, we selected the 156 female guardians who were caring for elderly female wards.

The female guardians ranged in age from 31 to 87 (M age = 59 years) and were most often married (61%) or widowed (22%). Family members held 67% of the guardianships (30%–adult daughters; 37%–other relatives), whereas 23% of the women were not related to their ward. Wards ranged in age from 63 to 104 with a mean age of 84 years. The majority of wards were widowed (59%) or never married (30%). Almost three-fourths of the wards resided in a nursing home or board and care facility.

Measures

In two of the three states studied, the courts require that guardians submit annual reports summarizing the activities and assistance they provide to their ward.[1] We coded these activities into the following ten categories: visit with the ward, provide emotional support, purchase personal items, file forms and complete paperwork, help with ADLs, prepare meals/food, take the ward to a physician, do laundry, shop with the ward, and take the ward to visit family.

Since court records provided little indication of ward-guardian interpersonal relationships, and in some states offered limited information about guardian activities, we sent questionnaires to guardians in each of the three states. The guardians provided information about their caregiving activities on behalf of the ward and their emotional reactions to the role as guardian. In addition to gathering background information about the guardian and ward, other areas examined were: proximity to the ward, the functional capacity of the ward, amount of contact and time spent on guardian activities, personal reflections on the role of guardian, advice for others and thoughts about aging, and role strain and difficulties of guardianship.

RESULTS

Guardianship Activities

The first annual reports filed by 58% of the women provided information about their activities as guardians (Table 1). Visiting with the ward was the dominant activity engaged in by guardians. More than one-half of the guardians reported that they provided emotional support to those for

---

1. In Colorado, courts did not require guardians to file annual reports, so there was no record of guardian activity in this state.

TABLE 1. Activities and Assistance Provided to Wards by Their Guardians

Assistance to Ward	N	Percentage
Visit with ward	45	83
Provide emotional support	30	58
Purchase personal items	22	42
File forms and complete paperwork	13	25
ADLs	8	15
Prepare meals/food	7	13
Do laundry	7	13
Take ward to physician	6	12
Shop with ward	6	11
Take ward to visit family	3	6

whom they cared. They provided less frequent instrumental assistance. For example, 42% of the guardians bought personal items for the ward and one-fourth completed forms and paperwork. The living arrangements of the wards and their needs for direct care shaped, at least in part, the type of relationship that wards and guardians maintained and the assistance the guardians provided. For example, guardians who undertook food preparation and laundry activities were more likely to be sharing a home with their wards than guardians who did not assume these activities.

Typology of Guardianship

How did these women respond to the legal caregiving role they assumed? We identified four patterns of guardianship based on guardians' written descriptions of the most difficult aspects of their roles and how they addressed the challenges. "Sympathetic" described the largest proportion of women (40%). These women focused on the needs of their wards and attended to the positive rather than negative aspects of their relationship. They were quite sensitive to the needs of others and emphasized wanting to do more for their wards, hoped they had made the most appropriate decisions in the best interests of their wards, and wanted assurance they were performing the best they could for those for whom they were responsible.

The second most frequent pattern was the "sad" (26%). These guardians highlighted the decline and suffering of the ward and the distressing visits with the ward. They seemed to suffer themselves as they observed the deterioration of their ward. They described the pain of their wards' decline, including the declaration of parents or close friends as incompetent.

The "challenged" (19%) were highly task-oriented as they addressed the needs of their wards. These guardians managed the available resources to ensure proper care for the ward, developed strategies for the protection of the ward, and advocated for the ward. They viewed solving multiple problems of the ward as a challenging and rewarding experience. The women acted with dispatch, stressing preparation and the use of resources to assist wards. The hallmarks of the challenged were feelings of competency and efficacy.

Guardians described as the "hostile" (15%) expressed negative feelings about guardianship. They made harsh judgments about most persons connected with the guardianship and toward the process. These guardians found the required paperwork distasteful and expressed hatred for and distrust of attorneys and the courts. Generally, guardianship was not to their liking, and it was not something they would undertake again.

Benefits of Guardianship

Despite their hardships, the majority of guardians also perceived benefits from and satisfaction with their position. The women described three types of benefits from being a legal caregiver: (a) the opportunity to help another, (b) personal gratification, and (c) protection of the financial and legal concerns of the ward. Some, however, found no positive features of guardianship.

The Opportunity to Help Others and Personal Gratification. The most frequent benefits of guardianship noted by the women were the opportunity to improve the care and the life of another (55%) and the personal gratification they felt from helping someone (24%). For some women, assuming the guardianship role allowed them the occasion to repay prior aid or favors received from the ward. Sometimes it was difficult to distinguish between personal gratification from service and gratitude for an opportunity to see to the best interests of the ward.

For several guardians, personal gratification satisfied feelings of wanting to be needed. Comments reflecting this feeling included: "Guardianship satisfies the altruistic needs of the guardian . . . and serves the community." "I felt good doing this (guardianship)." "You feel needed." Some wards were responsive to their guardians, and the latter benefited accordingly: "The ward's positive reactions to my visits were rewarding, especially when I brought my family." A positive response from a ward contrasted with experiences of guardians who believed their wards neither knew nor cared what they did for them.

Some women assessed their benefits with reference to the magnitude of the need. Illustrative comments were: "Feeling that I am meeting an important need and sometimes being able to protect the ward from exploitation." "The knowledge you are helping someone who can't help himself/herself is gratifying."

Some women viewed guardianship as the end of victimization. For example, one ward said, "It gives me peace of mind that the ward is being properly cared for and not in a position to be taken advantage of." Other guardians reported having peace of mind and a sense of closure about their ward's care. One older woman expressed her relief, "For me, I knew for sure my sister was being taken care of and loved." A 47 year old guardian commented, "I felt good knowing that I made her last four years of life a little better. She was my good friend and I loved her."

Included in the descriptions of gratification and beneficial outcomes were perceptions of equity and exchange. Serving as guardians provided the women the opportunity to repay a relative or friend for previously rendered services or help. One woman commented, "Earlier she gave me her best." Parents were often the recipients of the exchange. As one woman remarked, the greatest benefit was " . . . being with mom. She took care of me so I just returned her love." For some women, the hoped-for equity extended into the future. One woman noted, "I know my time is coming; I hope my kids will take care of me."

For other women, friendship was the focus of the exchange that crossed over time. Several of the women commented on how their care had benefited the wards:

> She is a very close friend and I didn't like to see her being treated as her children were treating her. This isn't happening now and physically she appears better.

> The ward had helped me years before, so I wanted to help her.

> The ward and I had been the best of friends for 20 years. She is very articulate and intelligent.

Thus, guardianship was an opportunity for some friends to reciprocate earlier assistance and to attain closure on a relationship. A 65 year old female guardian summarized it well, "I finally feel that I have been able to repay her (the ward) for her many kindnesses over the years. She really paid in advance for my help now."

Legal and Financial Oversight. Substantially fewer women perceived handling the legal and financial affairs of the ward as a primary benefit.

Keeping accurate records, paying bills on time, balancing bank accounts, and making prompt deposits were some legal activities conducted by the guardians. Safeguarding finances for personal care of the ward was important to guardians who cited legal and financial oversight as a special benefit. Others described more general advantages of their authority. For example, two benefits described by the guardians were the authority to advocate for persons who could not exercise their rights and that no one questioned their rights to act on behalf of the ward. One guardian summed up the advantages to her. She stated that the guardianship "provided stability in handling financial and legal matters. It provided continuity of care for the ward. It relieved other family members from worry."

The Absence of Benefits. Whereas some individuals experienced substantial benefits, other guardians were unable to mention any positive aspects of guardianship. A few of the women (12%) found nothing positive in their experience of caring for the ward. Those who could find no benefits to their role as guardians were outspoken in their negative views. For example, "There are no 'positives'!"; "It's an obligation to the ward, and I hate all of it!" Another summarized the advantages of having a guardianship as "None!" For some, the negative view was directed toward the process and requirements of guardianship when they believed they could accomplish the task of caring without the involvement of the court. For others, the hostility seemed focused on their displeasure with or perhaps even dislike of the ward.

Not surprising, few hostile guardians expressed personal gratification from their guardian activities (16%). Approximately one-fourth (26%) of the hostile did not see any benefits to having the guardianship in contrast to 7 to 10% of the other types.

Guardianship and Women's Views of Old Age

In what way did the role of legal caregiver shape the respondents' perceptions of aging in general as well as conceptions of their own future? Previous research on those who care for the aged often does not connect the caregiving experience with the caregivers' management or anticipation of their own aging. To consider the effect of guardianship on views of old age held by guardians, we examined the beliefs and values they used to organize their behavior and to interpret their experiences as a guardian with reference to their own aging. The interpretation of the guardianship experience shaped the sense of the future held by several women.

The sense of the future sometimes was one of gloom, often centering on the decline in the ward's condition and its implications for the guardian's own prospects. Guardians' views, of how guardianship had influenced the meaning of old age, illustrate several of Hasselkus's (1988) themes of meaning. For example, a sense of managing as exemplified in planning, a sense of fear and risk, and a sense of the future. In Hasselkus' research on caregivers, a sense of managing was a pervasive theme illustrated by feeling things were under control and a sense of getting things done. Among guardians, managing was the awareness of the need to plan and to prepare for old age. Hasselkus observed a sense of future among caregivers in which caregiving activities often included a pervasive perception of doom especially about the possible deteriorating condition of care recipients. As a parallel, guardians often expressed worries about a potentially bleak future when they grow old; caregiving heightened their worries. A sense of fear and risk among persons studied by Hasselkus referred to a fear of change or anything that might cause a change in the condition of the care recipient. Among guardians, a sense of fear or risk applied to their own well-being. For example, the possible deterioration of their health and the absence of someone to care for them if they should be in a condition similar to their ward were sources of fear for some.

Presumably, guardianship occurs only in instances of extreme vulnerability, either physical, mental, or functional. Consequently, guardians most often have contact with and responsibility for the aged with the greatest frailties. This experience with fragility undoubtedly influenced guardians' conceptions of aging.

We asked the women if being a guardian changed their thinking about old age. If their duties as a guardian had changed their views of later life, the women described the ways in which their thinking about old age had altered. Approximately one-half (54%) of the women agreed that guardianship had changed their perspective on old age. From their responses (see Table 2), we identified predominate ways in which they had come to regard old age.

Personal Concern and Worry. The largest proportion of women for whom guardianship had shaped their views of aging expressed worry and concern about their own aging and about what would happen to them. Their concerns about aging as an outcome of their guardianship experience focused on the hope and expectation that someone would be available to care for them, and an expression of a personal, but sometimes general fear of aging.

Expectation of Future Assistance. The women expressed their hope that if they needed help in the future, they would receive it. One woman age 45 said, "Mother was the fourth elderly person I cared for until death. I hope

TABLE 2. The Effects of Guardianship on Guardians' Views of Aging

Effect[a]	N	Percentage
Personal concern and worry	36	47
Concern for the aged	17	22
Awareness of the need to plan for old age	11	15
Importance of health and quality of life	6	8
Importance of social support	3	3
Resistance to aging	2	3

[a]Based on responses of 76 women who described how guardianship had affected their views of aging.

someone will be kind to me when and if I need it in my last years." Other women commented:

> I know my turn is coming and hope my kids take care of me.

> I hope that someone will be there to help me when I get old!

Some women had considered the possibility that no one would be available to help them should they need it. As illustrated by the following comments, such thoughts appeared linked to a fear of old age:

> What will happen to me if there is no one for me?

> Old age is frightening if your health is impaired. Who will take care of me? I hope I get as good care as my mom has.

In summary, some women with these views described exchanges they expected to receive from their children. Others who were more tentative and perhaps less sure of future assistance expressed the hope that someone would be available to help them.

Worry and Fear of Aging. The women also expressed more global concerns of worry and fear about aging. For example, one woman said, "Since I am 71 years old, it causes me to worry about my own future." A woman of 40 said, "Since being a guardian, old age scares me more." A guardian who was 52 years old commented, "It's more scary than I thought. I see the vulnerability." "Old age scares me silly," was a feeling noted by a 37 year old guardian.

Still others articulated more specific fears about possible correlates of aging. A 62 year old guardian revealed a specific fear, "I am afraid my personality will change." Another woman said, "I have been left with a fear of growing older and ending up that way (like the ward)." A 70 year old guardian noted, "I have become very aware of the last days of the elderly." The prospects of aging with the possibility of prolonged disability requiring residence in a nursing home or the threat of aging without support were some of the worries prompted by the experience of guardianship.

General Concerns for Older Persons as a Group. About one-fifth of the guardians expressed a greater awareness of the needs of the older population. They commented on the negative attitudes toward aging held by the public, the help older persons may need, and the sympathy they had developed for their elders. The women expressed their growing awareness about the circumstances of some of the aged. Younger guardians expressed these thoughts more often than older guardians. Unlike their earlier comments, they directed their views not toward their own aging but rather they reflected concern for the welfare of others as they coped with aging. Comments from several guardians illustrate their concerns:

> Since being a guardian I am far more concerned about older persons' well-being.

> I've learned that sometimes it's very hard to become old.

> Old people need more care and help than I realized in all aspects of their lives.

The women saw beyond the mechanism of guardianship and described the importance of affection and caring. For example, one woman said, "I saw how much an older person needs someone who loves them to watch over them and their care and welfare." Contact with their ward provided them insight into difficulties confronted by some older persons. Their observations were general and did not necessarily characterize persons for whom they cared, or reflect specifically on their own aging.

Awareness of the Need to Plan. Because of their guardianship, 15% of the women concluded they should begin to plan for old age. Guardianship had made them realize the importance of planning for later life. A 65 year old woman suggested, "Prepare–prepare–prepare!" Others commented:

> I am much more aware of the need to plan more carefully toward the day that I may need a guardian.

> It's better to get things in order before you get old.

The objectives of planning ranged from easing the burden for others to ensuring the completion of personal wishes. As one woman stated, "People should realize the importance of making their wishes known—such as living wills, what to do with family heirlooms, etc."

Some guardians provided specific reasons for their admonition to plan. As one woman said, "Observing Alzheimer's at close hand has made me realize I should prepare for this possibility myself." For some, the advice about planning was to avert an experience like that of the ward. For example, a 41 year old granddaughter said, "I will make a living will so as not to be put on life-sustaining equipment or a food tube as my grandmother is."

Importance of Health Maintenance and Social Support. Although several women expressed hope that assistance would be available for them, others discussed the importance of support more generally. For example, one women stated, "It's important, if at all possible, to have a trustworthy friend or relative." Eight percent said guardianship had made them think of the importance of health as an aspect of aging. The comment of a 57 year old guardian reflected the salience of health maintenance, "I will try to take care of myself and conscientiously try to be mentally alert."

Resignation and Resistance to Aging. A few women observed that the major impact of their activities as guardians was to make them want to avoid old age and to die early. The statements from three guardians illustrate these views:

> I don't particularly want to get there (old age).

> Die younger!

> Don't get old—especially if you have no family.

For most guardians who contemplated old age differently than before assuming their roles, it was the incapacity of their wards rather than the wards' age that influenced their thinking. Guardians explicitly or implicitly mentioned circumstances that may or may not accompany old age (i.e., illness, disability, and/or dependency). Thus, the guardians' changing perceptions of aging, in part, reflected a response to disability or incapacity. Others also suggested that people usually do not view aging per se as negatively as disability, which often relates to reduced expectations for growth, development, and decision making (Atchley, 1991).

Changed views of aging differed according to the typologies of guardianship. The largest percentage of guardians whose ideas about aging changed was the "hostile" (80%). Substantially fewer women (53-56%)

in the other patterns noted changes in their thoughts about aging since becoming a guardian. The hostile also were the least likely to indicate that the guardianship had caused them to worry more about themselves and their own aging (26%). In contrast, the "challenged" (75%) and the "sad" (53%) most often found the guardianship evoked worries about what would happen to them. The hostile were most likely to mention their increased awareness of the need to plan because of having been a guardian (33%). Ten percent or fewer of the other types described the need to plan as an outcome of their being a guardian.

IMPLICATIONS FOR PRACTICE AND FUTURE RESEARCH

Unlike informal caregiving, which has become a normative activity for many families, becoming and being a guardian is not a normative experience for most individuals. Although these women provided emotional and instrumental assistance to their wards as informal caregivers would, the guardianship relationship they had with their female wards had an additional influence on their lives. When deriving meaning from their role as guardians, some women were sympathetic to the needs of their ward or challenged by the instrumental tasks of managing a guardianship. Yet, others appeared saddened by or reacted with hostility to the whole process. Despite the different ways in which guardians derived meaning from their experience, the majority enjoyed benefits or satisfaction from their role, although a small percentage reported no positive benefits of being a guardian. The women who responded with hostility to the guardianship process raised questions of why they reacted so negatively and if such a negative reaction has any long term influence on perceptions of their aging. What is most apparent from the data is that a formalized role–that of being a guardian–had an affective outcome, both negative and positive, on those who occupied that role. This affective influence on guardians is surprising in that most did not provide traditional 24 hours a day, 7 days a week caregiving services. In spite of this difference, it appears that the process of obtaining a guardianship and carrying out the responsibilities of a guardian was not a benign experience. Since guardianships are for the very frail and vulnerable, guardians must cope with managing the lives of the very dependent.

Many guardians were not adult children, but rather a sibling or more distant relative (e.g., a niece) or a friend of the ward. Guardians often felt compelled to take on the formal caregiving role because of the history of their relationship with the ward. In the instances where guardians and wards have been friends for many years, one wonders how the relationship between the guardian and ward changes with the advent of their friend's physical and mental impairment as well as the role changes a guardianship formalizes. There is some evidence to suggest that friendships do change over time with the advent of changes in personal health (Johnson & Troll, 1994; Roberto, 1993), but there is little empirical information about the changing relationship between guardians and wards. Investigations that include more in-depth data regarding the past and current relationship from both members of the dyad (when possible) would provide greater insight into how wards and guardians adjust to the inequalities of the guardian-ward relationship.

REFERENCES

Atchley, R. (1991). *Social forces and aging.* Belmont, CA: Wadsworth.

Bulcroft, K., Kielkopf, M., & Tripp, K. (1991). Elderly wards and their legal guardians: Analysis of county probate court records in Ohio and Washington. *The Gerontologist, 31,* 156-164.

Clipp, E., & George, L. (1990). Caregiver needs and patterns of social support. *Journals of Gerontology, 45,* S102-S111.

Dwyer, J., & Coward, R. (1992). Gender, family, and long-term care of the elderly. In J. Dwyer & R. Coward (Eds.), *Gender, families, and eldercare* (pp. 3-17). Newbury Park, CA: Sage.

Hasselkus, B. (1988). Meaning in family caregiving: Perspectives on caregiver/professional relationships. *The Gerontologist, 28,* 686-691.

Hommel, P., Wang, L., & Bergman, J. (1990). Trends in guardianship reform: Implications for the medical and legal professions. *Law, Medicine and Health Care, 18,* 213-226.

Johnson, C. & Troll, L. (1994). Constraints and facilitators to friendships in late late life. *The Gerontologist, 34,* 79-87.

Keith, P. M., & Wacker, R. R. (1994). *Older wards and their guardians.* New York: Praeger.

Pearlin, L., Mullan, J., Semple, S., & Skaff, M. (1990). Caregiving and the stress process: An overview of concepts and their measures. *The Gerontologist, 30,* 583-594.

Roberto, K. A. (1993). *Friendships of older women: Changes over time.* Final report to the Henry A. Murray Research Center, Radcliffe College. Greeley, CO: University of Northern Colorado, Gerontology Program.

Scharlach, A., & Boyd, S. (1989). Caregiving and employment: Results of an employee survey. *The Gerontologist, 29,* 382-387.

Stone, R., Cafferata, G., & Sangl, J. (1987). Caregivers of the frail elderly: A national profile. *The Gerontologist, 27,* 616-626.

Walker, A., Martin, S., & Jones, L. (1992). Benefits and costs of caregiving and care receiving for daughters and mothers. *Journals of Gerontology: Social Sciences, 47,* S130-S139.

Zarit, G., Todd, P., & Zarit, J. (1986). Subjective burden of husbands and wives as caregivers: A longitudinal study. *The Gerontologist, 26,* 260-266.

Older Women
Living in a Continuing Care
Retirement Community:
Marital Status and Friendship Formation

Margaret A. Perkinson, PhD
David D. Rockemann, MS

SUMMARY. Ethnographic observations and interviews with twenty female residents of a new Continuing Care Retirement Community (CCRC) revealed the patterns of friendship development experienced by older women. Qualitative analyses identified various phases of friendship development and aspects of the social context that facilitated friendship formation in its earliest stages. Marital status was a major factor in the selection of friends within this setting. Friendship styles and strategies for developing friendships varied considerably. Although most women successfully formed new friendships within this setting, certain subgroups seemed at risk for social isolation. *[Article copies available from The Haworth Document Delivery Service: 1-800-342-9678. E-mail address: getinfo@haworth.com]*

Residents of age-homogeneous settings, such as retirement communities, experience higher rates of social interaction and higher levels of

---

Margaret A. Perkinson is Senior Research Scientist, Polish Research Institute, Philadelphia Geriatric Center, Philadelphia, PA 19141.

David D. Rockemann is Administrator of Health Care Services, Riddle Village, Media, PA 19063.

[Haworth co-indexing entry note]: "Older Women Living in a Continuing Care Retirement Communty: Marital Status and Friendship Formation." Perkinson, Margaret A. and David D. Rockemann. Co-published simultaneously in the *Journal of Women & Aging* (The Haworth Press, Inc.) Vol. 8, Nos. 3/4, 1996, pp. 159-177; and: *Relationships Between Women in Later Life* (ed: Karen A. Roberto) The Haworth Press, Inc., 1996, pp. 159-177; and: *Relationships Between Women in Later Life* (ed: Karen A. Roberto) Harrington Park Press, an imprint of The Haworth Press, Inc., 1996, pp. 159-177. [Single or multiple copies of this article are available from the Haworth Document Delivery Service: 1-800-342-9678, 9:00 a.m. - 5:00 p.m. (EST). E-mail address: getinfo@haworth.com] social integration and morale than older adults who live in age-integrated settings (Bultena, 1974; Lawton, 1970; Rosow, 1967). Ethnographic studies (Perkinson, 1980, 1995; Ross, 1977) indicate that this increased social interaction encourages the development of a sense of community, social support, new roles and normative systems. Studies of social ties in retirement communities and other age-segregated housing suggest that friendships flourish for many residents (Adams, 1986; Shea, Thompson, & Blieszner, 1988; Stacey-Konnert & Pynoos, 1992). Shea et al. (1988) suggest that age density, frequent contact among residents, and the "leveling effect" (whereby individuals deem past social distinctions as irrelevant) are factors that contribute to the development of new friendships. Age-homogeneous settings seem to exert a greater impact on older women than on older men. Women show greater increases in social activity and involvement in friendships (Rosow, 1967; Silverman, 1987), perhaps because they outnumber men in these settings and thus have larger pools of potential friends from which to choose.

While Adams' (1986) study of friendships among older women suggests that age-segregated settings enhance the development of emotionally close ties, others disagree. Shea et al. (1988) examined the friendships predominantly between females in a newly opened retirement community. They compared residents' patterns of resource exchange with their previous friends and with friends recently made in the retirement community. They found significant differences in patterns of sharing information or advice. Although residents engaged in intimate self-disclosures with their old friends, information exchanged with their new retirement community friends typically consisted of conversations on daily events or other impersonal topics. Stacey-Konnert and Pynoos (1992) found a similar pattern in their sample of continuing care retirement community (CCRC) residents, 80% of whom were women. Residents maintained confidant relationships with old friends who lived outside the CCRC or with CCRC friends who were also pre-move friends of long-standing. Although new friendships did develop within the CCRC, intimate confidant relationships were generally limited to those friends who had shared a long history of experiences.

There clearly are variations in friendship development, even within such seemingly homogeneous populations as residents of age-homogeneous settings. Stacey-Konnert and Pynoos (1992) identified various types of residents who were less socially integrated and experienced greater difficulty establishing friendships: those with declining physical or mental health, caregivers, the very old, and social isolates. Rockemann and Perkinson (1993) demonstrated that residents who had moved to a CCRC from the local area tended to maintain their involvement in the outside community, and were less involved than non-local residents in activities and relationships within the retirement community.

Marital status represents another important factor affecting friendship selection and maintenance (Lopata, 1979). A change in marital status can result in significant changes in friendship networks (Allan & Adams, 1989). Married women tend to disengage from widowed friends for a variety of reasons (Lopata, 1975), and widows become more involved with other widows. The social context in which this takes place strongly influences this process (Blau, 1961), as seen within age-homogeneous settings with high concentrations of widows (Petrowsky, 1976; Stacey-Konnert & Pynoos, 1992).

In this paper we focus on the impact of social context on the process of friendship formation among female residents of a newly developed CCRC. We first outline the trajectory of friendship development as experienced by our respondents, and describe the impact of the age-homogeneous context on various phases of friendship formation. We then focus on marital status as a major criterion the women used in selecting friends within this community, and on the emerging social groups and divisions that resulted. Throughout the discussion, we note variation in strategies for developing friends and differences in friendship styles.

METHOD

The Sample

The sample consisted of 20 female Riverdale Village residents, selected based on marital status as part of a quota sampling. Equal numbers of married non-caregivers, widows, and never-marrieds were randomly selected from a master list of residents. Spousal caregivers were selected from a list compiled by the CCRC's nursing staff. The ages of the women ranged from 71 to 92 (M = 78). All but two women had lived in the CCRC from 12 to 20 months. All but three women had moved to Riverdale Village from the local area, and had lived in this area for most of their adult lives. The women were well-educated; eleven (55%) were high school graduates, one (5%) attended junior college, and eight (40%) graduated from college.

Data Collection

The two authors tape-recorded and transcribed all interviews. Interviews lasted approximately 90 minutes to two hours. Besides answering basic demographic and background questions, the women identified their best friends (including CCRC residents and/or non-residents); identified their closest friends within Riverdale Village and the activities they shared; identified any Riverdale Village activities and informal groups in which they participated; described any services they used; and discussed their thoughts about friendship in later life, comparing their Riverdale Village friendships to those made before their move. At the end of the interview the women could also include additional observations about friendships within the CCRC and factors influencing friendship formation.

We reviewed and coded all transcripts. Using a grounded theory approach (Schatzman & Strauss, 1973; Strauss, 1987), we identified underlying themes and patterns, and selected various quotes from the women to illustrate them. Observations of social interactions within public areas (e.g., the dining rooms and lobbies) supplemented interviews, confirming and providing greater insight into social phenomena described by the women, such as the informal evening discussion groups and the various cliques.

THE SETTING

At the time of data collection, Riverdale Village was a 20-month old CCRC, located in a medium-sized town in southeastern Pennsylvania on a 40-acre campus adjacent to a community hospital. Its independent living section housed 305 residents ranging from 60 to 95 years old. Its skilled nursing facility and the assisted living facility were still under construction, requiring the relocation of 12 frail residents to neighboring nursing homes. A variety of structured activities provided abundant opportunities for residents to meet and interact with other residents. Residents also regularly gathered in informal groups in various public spaces, such as the game rooms or the lobbies.

FINDINGS

During the brief time Riverdale Village had been opened, most women had developed friendships with other residents. However, the majority said their best friends lived outside the CCRC. Two of the twenty women admitted all their best friends had died. Of the remaining 18 women, 13 (72%) reported all their closest friends lived outside Riverdale Village. Two (11%) maintained close friendships with both Riverdale Village residents and with people outside the CCRC. The remaining three (17%) said all their closest friends were Riverdale Village residents. The minority of

Riverdale Village residents who maintained close friendships within the CCRC tended to fall into two categories. They were either very old women (in their 90's) who were unable to maintain past friendships because of the death or frailty of former close friends, or they were women whose closest friends had also moved to Riverdale Village.

The Trajectory of Friendship Formation

First encounters. Most women had moved to Riverdale from the surrounding area. As one woman remarked, "We used to say half of Rockville moved in here, so there are a lot of people that I know of and have now made as friends."

Although they may not have known many residents when first moving into the CCRC, most of the women who came from the local community soon found they shared much in common with their new neighbors. An 81 year old never-married respondent explained:

> You find as time goes on in talking to people you find people that you can relate to. You have similar backgrounds and they know similar people that you knew. And they came from similar neighborhoods that you know of. I found people here that I knew or that knew similar things that I knew.

Observant fellow residents who recognized common bonds often introduced newcomers to potential friends. Two never-married women described how they first met their best friends at Riverdale Village:

> When I just got here of course I didn't know anyone, but somebody introduced me to Gale who's also from Delaware, so that sort of broke the ice there. And then we gravitated toward each other . . .

> It's strange to say, she lived on the same street for many years that I did in Haventown, but it was a busy street and you couldn't even call across to the neighbors, and she lived a whole block down. The only thing I knew about her was she loved her garden. She has become perhaps the closest friend I have here . . . I think I met her on the first night . . . Somebody came up to me and said, "Didn't you live on Drex Avenue?" and I said, "Yes." She said, "I think your neighbor who lived on Drex is your neighbor now here," and they introduced me to her.

The communal nature of life in the CCRC offered easy access to new acquaintances and many opportunities for social interaction for those who wanted it. Occasions for meeting fellow residents ranged from highly formal occasions organized by the CCRC staff to facilitate friendship formation, such as the wine and cheese parties, to impromptu gatherings around the community jigsaw puzzle table when people briefly stopped to chat and add a few pieces to the puzzle currently in progress. Some residents, such as an 83 year old married respondent, literally opened their homes to their neighbors, encouraging spontaneous informal visiting analogous to college dormitory life:

> Well, they just come in maybe for a sandwich. Mary walked by and then I said, "Oh look, my neighbor just brought me a whole big dish of tuna fish, how about coming in and having a sandwich." That's what happens to us, our neighbors are just fabulous . . . yeah, come back and forth, oh, they're nice, my neighbors, just great they are.

Establishing mutual interests. People with similar interests often found each other through their involvement in various Riverdale Village activities. A married respondent explained:

> You get to know people depending on what you do. If you exercise, you get to know the exercise group. Now I'm in arts and crafts, so I know a lot more people because I work with them. And then I'm on the decorating committee, so there are other people that work on that that I get to know. It's involvement with different activities.

Evening meals represented opportunities to interact with the greatest variety of residents. If compatible dining partners identified common interests, they could easily arrange to pursue them, thus opening the possibility for further friendship development. The women frequently mentioned playing cards, especially bridge, as a context for continued interaction with potential friends. One woman described the development of her closest friendship within Riverdale Village:

> That's how we met, at dinner one Sunday. I remember when I met Sarah, and, "Oh, you play bridge," and then she knew someone else who played bridge, and then we just got together and played bridge . . . During the week we just decide if we have nothing else to do we would meet and play bridge or even pinochle . . .

Validation of friendship status. In general, the women could quickly assess the compatibility of a potential companion. One 70 year old married informant described this reaction as, "A short click in the beginning, and you see more and more of each other."

Nevertheless, most recognized that solid friendships evolved over time, through a history of shared experiences and confidences:

> Friendships are the things that develop. I don't feel you can force it and say you are going to be my good friend. I think you can be friendly with a lot of people, but a really close friendship has to develop over time.

Requests for special favors or help sometimes signified the transition in a relationship from acquaintance to friend, since the person in need was forced to identify the individual on whom she could rely. The comments of one respondent illustrate such a transition:

> I felt very good the other day when she had a young man come put some appliance on her to stretch her neck. She called and said would I come up while he was doing this because her husband was going to be out. She said, "I don't know who else to ask." I said, "I'm so glad you did, what are friends for if you don't help each other?"

Residents reinforced friendships with various types of exchange. Those who continued to drive offered rides shopping or to church to those who had given up their cars. A neighbor might watch another's apartment while that friend was in the hospital. Some pairs of friends engaged in frequent exchanges of food, as one never-married respondent described:

> The Jones sisters and I will buy a thing of celery together, because when you only cook one meal a day, it goes bad. So I buy the celery and they take one. I gave them rice pudding, and they gave me some homemade German potato salad. And they're in my building and that makes it easier. So we have lots of little things like that.

On the other hand, some residents felt keen disappointment when expected support did not materialize, indicating that a presumed friendship was not mutual. One widow, confined to her room for health reasons, revealed:

> I kind of thought that people here would be more sympathetic to the cause, so to speak. That they would have come up, say, "Rita, do you need anything at the store?" or "Rita, is there anything I can do to help you?" And that didn't happen.

The evening meal as social crucible. The evening meal represented a setting of special significance for both friendship development and social exclusion within the CCRC. The various groupings of diners signified a daily display of current friendship alliances and dissolutions for all to see. Residents noted the cliques, the loners, the socially gracious and amiable, and those who battled openly in this most public arena.

By observing an individual's public behavior in the dining rooms, residents could evaluate that person from afar. One widowed respondent explained how she ruled out certain people as potential friends, based on their actions at mealtime:

> Like in the dining room, you can tell a lot about people. A lot of people are very short and inconsiderate of the waiters, and that I cannot abide. So when I find somebody like that, I think, I don't want to get too close to them, 'cause I don't like that. You prejudge, but then that's the only way you can do sometimes, prejudging somebody to see how they talk to what they consider are people working for them.

An unpleasant exchange with a dining partner was sufficient cause to eliminate him/her from the pool of potential friends. A never-married respondent described past dining encounters and the various criteria she used in assessing dining companions:

> I like a person who is not too critical. Sometimes I've eaten with people here and they criticize every blessed thing, the food, everything, or they're too loud. Or I should say, too aggressive maybe in mannerisms.

Many residents viewed their dining time as an opportunity to meet new people and develop new friends. One married respondent described her dining strategy:

> We always eat with different people. We do what we call "Riverdale Roulette" in the dining room. And you go in and you either start a table or finish a table. And that way you get to meet a lot of people.

Other residents settled into a routine of eating with the same people every evening and lost the opportunity to expand their friendship networks. A married woman described her dining pattern:

> My husband and I eat with four other women. We've kind of settled into eating, a routine of eating at a six-top table in the Chesapeake Room every night, which I guess limits friendships, because you're not sitting with other couples all the time.

Some dining groups were more "permeable" than others (i.e., more receptive to including additional residents). A married respondent described her "open group" of dining partners:

> The three of us, we eat all the time together. But if we can get a table for others, we prefer to have somebody, yeah we break up, we have somebody 'cause that's the only way you get to meet people.

Many residents criticized the more exclusive dining groups. For example, one never-married respondent and her sister had eaten with the same widowed neighbor every night since their first evening at Riverdale Village. Over time their group expanded to include four additional widows:

> We get a table for seven when we can get one, or otherwise we split three and four or whatever we get. And they usually place us at tables side by side. We make a lot of noise in the dining room . . . Some people think we are too close . . . Some people have said it is nice to eat with other people at night and get to learn more people that way. We seem to get around more than most people anyway. When they split the table up, no one else joins us. There is still the three and four to make seven.

Marital Status as a Major Criterion for Friendship Selection

Consonant with other research findings on the influence of marital status on social relations (Brown, 1975; Lopata, 1975; Stacey-Konnert & Pynoos, 1992), marital status clearly exerted a major impact on women's friendship patterns within the CCRC. When we asked the women to identify their closest friends in Riverdale Village, singles (i.e., widows and never-marrieds) invariably mentioned other singles, and married women who were not caregivers mentioned other marrieds. There were strikingly few exceptions. One never-married respondent included one couple (the husband had been a life-long family friend) among her friends; two married non-caregivers included one widow as a friend (both also had been life-long friends). Married women who were active caregivers for their husbands represented an interesting exception. Of those who had friends in the CCRC, all but one included both marrieds and widows among their closest Riverdale Village friends. It appeared that caregiving represented a transitional stage in friendship development within this CCRC, a period when women may alter their association patterns and shift reference groups.

The married non-caregivers. The impact of marital status was not limited to the choice of closest friends, but extended to CCRC friendship patterns in general. There was a distinct social division between married and non-married women. Most accepted this situation, as one widowed respondent remarked:

> You find that here, a lot of couples stick together and a lot of single ladies stick together. I guess that's normal . . . I am friendly with some ladies that are still with a spouse, but the rest of them tend to keep together, which is fine. They have more in common.

Single and married women had different theories to explain this social division. The widow just quoted suggested that husbands limited married residents' involvement with others:

> A lot of ladies I think would like to do things with the single ladies, but they really can't. They're really tied . . . That's what I've observed . . . I'll say, "Well, why don't we do so and so? and "Why aren't you on that list?" "Well, he doesn't want to," or "I can't leave him," or "I have to take him to the doctor." So it's a little different.

A married respondent offered a different perspective:

> We do have some widow friends, just a few, I haven't mentioned. It's more pleasant really if you're coupled to be with couples. It's not great for the man to be with a lot of widowed ladies. Besides, they might make a pass at him.

The "threat" of the unattached woman has surfaced in other studies (Lopata, 1979), and reflects a common assumption among older adults that cross-sex friendships invariably involve an erotic element (Adams, 1985; Wright, 1989).

The personal characteristics of a husband and his level of involvement in the social world of Riverdale Village either hindered or facilitated his wife's social involvement. Many men preferred to indulge in their own pursuits in the privacy of their apartments rather than engage in the various informal groups (composed mainly of women) that met in the lobby after dinner. Many women chose to accompany their husbands rather than join the groups alone:

> My husband usually makes a "bee-line" for the television and the baseball game. I stay with him. I don't seem to be inclined to get involved in activities without him.

Some men could not participate in group activities for various reasons. A 91 year old respondent admitted that she discontinued her association with one informal evening group because of her husband's discomfort:

> My husband is hard of hearing, but he does have a hearing aide. But when he gets in a group, this is a fairly large group in the (lobby), and he is surrounded, he has a hard time . . . I would go with the group. He would stay for a while, then he would go up to the apartment, because a lot of the conversation he couldn't catch. And it's embarrassing to him because he has never been handicapped that way.

Other men spent most of their time outside Riverdale Village. The husband of one woman continued to work full-time, and played tennis three or four times a week with a friend outside the CCRC (missing dinner and the opportunity to interact with other residents in the process). His wife was essentially free to spend her time as she pleased, and was one of the most actively involved of all the women in Riverdale Village activities and friendships. In contrast, another husband actively engaged in Riverdale groups and activities:

> He's floor representative to the Resident Association. He's in the chess club. He's on the newspaper, he does a lot of writing on that . . . He's been working on recycling projects . . .

This man met other residents through his various activities. As he introduced them to his wife, her social network expanded accordingly.

Married women sometimes chose friends within Riverdale Village based on the potential compatibilities of their husbands. As one woman reported, "When you're married, you have to consider the husband or mate, match the friendships on that side."

Spousal caregivers. As noted in other studies of friendship patterns in retirement communities (Stacey-Konnert & Pynoos, 1992), providing care for an impaired spouse limited opportunities to develop and maintain friendships within the CCRC. Many caregiving respondents skipped Riverdale Village activities to stay at home with their husbands. When asked whether she attended various CCRC events or activities, one woman replied:

> I haven't gone to any of that. I'd like to, but I don't like to leave my husband by himself. He's blind and he gets around, but not the way I'd like to see him.

Older caregivers admitted that they preferred to focus their time and energy on their spouses rather than starting new friendships. As one caregiver said, "I spend more time with my husband. I feel we have little time together at our age."

Caregivers of dementia patients spoke of their discomfort in the CCRC's dining room, especially if their spouse was unable to converse or to feed himself. Some chose to dine early and limited themselves to tables for two, thus avoiding unpleasant encounters, but also avoiding opportunities to develop relationships with sympathetic residents. Others gradually identified empathetic residents and attempted to join other tables:

> I guess I'm a little hesitant to get involved with people that can't understand why George doesn't enter into the conversation. Somebody told me that was ridiculous, not to worry about something like that. And I think that it's easy for them to say, but it's hard for me to do sometimes. As more and more people have gotten to know me, and understand that George isn't going to chatter away at the table and it doesn't bother them, then I'm less reluctant to go down and sit with other people.

There was surprisingly little peer support among Riverdale Village caregivers. The caregivers in our sample did not include other caregivers among their closest friends. Few admitted even knowing other residents who provided care for a spouse. This represents a sharp contrast to the social dynamics of caregiving found in an older and much larger CCRC (Perkinson, 1995), in which resident caregivers had developed an extensive system of mutual support. A "culture of caregiving" had evolved in this older setting, with residents sharing caregiving strategies and negotiating shared definitions of "appropriate" caregiving behavior. In Riverdale Village, on the other hand, there was a real reluctance to talk about caregiving experiences. This taboo prevented caregiving spouses from identifying each other and exchanging information and support. When asked whether she knew any other women within Riverdale Village who were taking care of their spouse, one caregiver answered:

> I don't think I do. I know there are people that I have met whose husbands are incapacitated, but I don't know to what extent they take care of their husbands. It's not something that people talk about in general.

Another caregiving respondent admitted she discussed her experiences with caregivers outside Riverdale Village, but not with CCRC caregivers:

> Yes, with a support group on the outside. We shared a lot of the same things. But not recently—not here. That was before we moved here.

The absence of self-disclosure and confiding among Riverdale Village caregivers may relate to the age of the CCRC and the general stage of friendship development that characterized most relationships within the community. One caregiver explained:

> They are more like acquaintances. I have not been involved in their life yet. I'm sure in time if you're here long enough and they're here long enough, you will become friends. But in a year you are only an acquaintance. You would not tell a person very personal things, to people you had just met.

Also, persons caring for spouses in the initial stages of infirmity often attempt to "cover up" for the spouse to maintain an image of health and well-being for as long as possible (Blum, 1991). This occurred even among new caregivers in the more established CCRC described above (Perkinson, 1995). All Riverdale Village residents were relatively recent move-ins. Perhaps emergent signs of disability provoked the move for some. These couples were neither ready nor willing to publicly admit their situation, especially among strangers and in a context in which staff had not yet clearly articulated the procedures and criteria for moving to higher levels of care (i.e., to the assisted living facility or the nursing home still under construction).

While Riverdale caregivers did not exchange support with each other, some did turn to residents who clearly identified themselves as former caregivers, i.e., the widows. One woman described the help she received:

> I don't know anyone who's doing it (caregiving) right now, but in talking with them, talking with (the widows) here, it's just a pattern. They're the survivors, they took care of their husband. And they will share some of their experiences with you. Some are private, but they are supportive because they know what you're going through . . . They recognize that you can get tired; they empathize with the things that are happening to you because they've been through it . . . They have offered to come and relieve me, you know, to sit with me. They've offered supplies, wheelchairs, whatever.

As noted earlier, married caregivers were the only group of women who consistently identified both married and single women among their closest Riverdale friends. Caregiving might represent a transitional status within this community where marital status so strongly influenced relationship development. As a husband declined in health and functional status, he was less able to maintain his role in the social world of couples, both as a companion to his wife and companion to the husbands of his wife's friends. As caregiving demands increased, the wife often disengaged from planned activities and informal groups, as noted above.

However, if the caregiving career progressed to the point where the husband moved to the nursing home, the caregiving wife was free to re-engage in community life. For example, one nursing home caregiver re-entering the social world of the CCRC found herself transformed into the social equivalent of a single woman. This transformation had significant implications for friendship development and maintenance, as the case of one respondent whose husband resided in an outside nursing home clearly illustrates (Since the nursing home at Riverdale Village was under construction at the time of data collection, residents who required skilled nursing care temporarily moved to neighboring facilities). This woman no longer felt welcome among married couples, a situation she accepted as natural:

> Well, it's just a normal thing. For instance, when you go to eat. You very rarely get to eat with couples, because they want another couple, which is understandable, because it makes an odd person at the table, unless there are two of you. But that's just a normal thing that happens in life.

After her daily lunchtime visit with her husband in the neighboring facility, she was free of caregiving responsibilities for the rest of the day. She socialized with her single friends, often at informal gatherings before dinner:

> Different groups, like they'll have four or five for a glass of wine or something, and then eat together, and I do that. Anytime anybody asks me or I have company, why you do that. And that's usually when it's all women, 'cause the couples, which is a normal reaction, are together. And that would have been the same for me if my husband hadn't been ill.

Her closest friend at Riverdale was a widow, with whom she spent considerable time:

> We just seem to get along and she was helpful to me. Sometimes when I wanted something and she was going to the store, she took

me a couple of times. Just, you know, how you get friendly with . . . And I was like a widow in a way and she was a widow. And we played bridge together.

However, the friendship lost its intensity when her widowed friend re-married. She explained:

We used to talk early in the morning. We used to eat together in the evening. But now she has a husband. It makes a slight difference. It's not like a single person when you have a husband. That's what I mean. We are still friendly, I don't mean that . . .

She felt little camaraderie with other caregivers in the community, since she regarded herself as a "married widow":

No, I'm not friendly with anyone who does (provide care for a spouse). They would be couples, and I'm not that intimate with couples. You don't get the opportunity . . . 'cause they're with their husbands and that makes a difference. I have found that out.

Widows and never-marrieds. Residents whose husbands died were clearly single again, and may have felt less ambivalence about their social status within the community. One married non-caregiver described the social transformation of several recent widows in Riverdale Village:

There are at least three women in here that I have seen who have blossomed since their husbands died. They were caregivers and had quite a responsibility and their husbands died and they got rid of the problem. And oh boy, they blossomed and they were out playing cards at night and they're having a wonderful time. It's sad, but it's great that they are back into the community and doing things . . .

Although some widows in the community appeared "socially rehabilitated," the widows interviewed were older and most suffered significant health or vision problems. Healthy residents often avoided their less active neighbors. One lively 83 year old married woman described a clique of frail older women and her interactions with them:

There's a bunch of ladies, all grouped together. They're all around the same age, they are all a little bit on the wobbly side, and they eat together. But I haven't been in contact with any of them closely. I'll say hello, grab their hand, every one of them, but that's about as close as I get to them. I like to be on the run, if you want to know the truth.

The two most frail widowed women spent most of the time confined in their rooms. One of them described her social isolation:

I don't have any friends at Riverdale Village . . . We have cliques here, these people are friendly, and these people are friendly, and these people are friendly, down the line. And if you're not in their little group or their clique, they can walk down the hall and not even speak to you.

The never-marrieds seemed more socially integrated than the widows in our sample. They all listed several never-married and widowed residents as friends, and were involved in various Riverdale Village activities and informal groups. Friendships may have held special significance for this group of women, as one never-married respondent explained:

I think as you get older, you're away from your family or your family's no longer living, and more people are seeking friendships. I mean, they don't have to be buddy-buddies, but they're somebody you can talk to . . . Because if you don't have any relatives and you get sick, who's going to look after you, just every day—not needs, because somebody's going to take care of your needs, but somebody to talk to.

CONCLUSIONS AND IMPLICATIONS

This age-homogeneous environment facilitated friendship formation by providing a large pool of potential friends (i.e., many women at the same stage of life who shared similar backgrounds and experiences). The abundance of public spaces and the generally public nature of life in the CCRC allowed residents to observe each other "from afar," to identify potential friends and eliminate others who appeared incompatible based on their public comportment. The communal evening meals and informal women's groups facilitated initial encounters. Structured activities allowed opportunities for sustained contact and interaction among women sharing common interests.

Nevertheless, many women described their relationships within the CCRC as acquaintances, with a potential for future development. This is undoubtedly because Riverdale Village was a "young" CCRC, in operation only 20 months. The dynamics of social interactions within an age-homogeneous setting are highly dependent on the age of the community, whether its residents are all newcomers and relative strangers to each other, or whether residents have lived in the setting for years and developed histories of shared experiences, complex networks, and strong ties of mutual support. Gross comparisons of age-segregated and age-integrated settings may be misleading if researchers do not account for this variation.

Research

We examined the ways in which various qualities of the social context of an age-homogeneous environment facilitated the process of friendship formation in its early stages. Suggestions for future research include: (a) studying the process of friendship formation over time; (b) exploring how social context affects the development, maintenance, and possible dissolution of relationships; and (c) observing how the formation of friendships affects the social context of the setting (e.g., what social divisions, networks, shared culture and traditions develop).

Practice

We noted considerable variation among the women in their strategies for developing friendships and their friendship styles. Most women seemed to adjust, and indeed, thrive as they developed social bonds within the community. Certain types of residents, however, had difficulties, and might benefit from special attention from staff in comparable settings. Several women identified themselves as "private persons," and faced a real dilemma in their attempts to preserve that privacy in such a communal, public setting. We noted various "distancing mechanisms," such as the development of cliques to exclude certain others and the "Riverdale Roulette" strategy of constantly changing dining partners to avoid spending significant amounts of time with any one person. Although administrators and staff often discourage such mechanisms in these settings, they may serve important functions for certain residents who are socially "overwhelmed" in their attempts to adjust to a more communal life-style.

We found that marital status represented an important factor in friendship formation within this setting, and spousal caregivers and widows were in especially vulnerable social positions. Staff and administrators should not assume that informal support systems composed of caregiving wives or widows will emerge spontaneously, especially in new age-segregated settings in which a sense of community is still developing. Formal support groups may provide a mechanism for these women to identify and interact with each other. Such formally organized groups may trigger the development of more informal peer counseling and support on a community-wide basis.

REFERENCES

Adams, R. (1985). Normative barriers to cross-sex friendships for elderly women. *The Gerontologist, 25,* 605-611.

Adams, R. (1986). Emotional closeness and physical distances between friends: Implications for elderly women living in age-segregated and age-integrated settings. *International Journal of Aging and Human Development, 22,* 55-74.

Allan, G. & Adams, R. (1989). Aging and the structure of friendship. In R. Adams & R. Blieszner (Eds.), *Older adult friendship* (pp. 45-64). Newbury Park, CA: Sage.

Blau, Z. (1961). Structural constraints on friendships in old age. *American Sociological Review, 26,* 429-439.

Blum, N. (1991). The management of stigma by Alzheimer family caregivers. *Journal of Contemporary Ethnography, 20,* 539-543.

Brown, B. (1975). A life-span approach to friendship: Age-related dimensions of an ageless relationship. In H. Lopata & D. Maines (Eds.), *Friendships in context* (pp. 23-50). Greenwich, CT: JAI Press.

Bultena, G. (1974). Structural effects on the morale of the aged: A comparison of age-segregated and age-integrated communities. In J. Gubrium (Ed.), *Late life communities and environmental policy* (pp. 18-31). Springfield, IL: Charles C. Thomas.

Lawton, M. P. (1970). Assessment, integration and environments for older people. *The Gerontologist, 10,* 38-46.

Lopata, H. (1975). Couple-companionate relationships in marriage and widowhood. In Nona Glazer-Malbin (Ed.), *Old family/new family* (pp. 119-149). New York: D. Van Nostrand Co.

Lopata, H. (1979). *Women as widows.* New York: Elsevier North Holland, Inc.

Perkinson, M. A. (1980). Alternate roles for the elderly: An example from a midwestern retirement community. *Human Organization, 39,* 219-226.

Perkinson, M. A. (1995). Socialization to the family caregiving role within a continuing care retirement community. *Medical Anthropology, 16,* 249-267.

Petrowsky, M. (1976). Marital status, sex and the social networks of the elderly. *Journal of Marriage and the Family, 38,* 749-756.

Rockemann, D. D. & Perkinson, M. A. (1993, July). *The effects of previous residence patterns on social integration within a CCRC.* Paper presented at the XVth meeting of the International Association of Gerontology, Budapest, Hungary.

Rosow, I. (1967). *Social integration of the aged.* New York: Free Press.

Ross, J. K. (1977). *Old people, new lives.* Chicago: University of Chicago Press.

Schatzman, L., & Strauss, A. (1973). *Field research: Strategies for a natural sociology.* Englewood Cliff, NJ: Prentice Hall.

Shea, L., Thompson, L., & Blieszner, R. (1988). Resources in older adults' old and new friendships. *Journal of Social and Personal Relationships, 5,* 83-96.

Silverman, P. (1987). Community settings. In P. Silverman (Ed.), *The elderly as modern pioneers* (pp. 234-262). Bloomington, IN: Indiana University Press.

Stacey-Konnert, C., & Pynoos, J. (1992). Friendship and social networks in a continuing care retirement community. *Journal of Applied Gerontology, 11,* 298-313.

Strauss, A. (1987). *Qualitative analysis for social scientists.* Cambridge: Cambridge University Press.

Wright, P. (1989). Gender differences in adults' same- and cross-gender friendships. In R. Adams & R. Blieszner (Eds.), *Older adult friendship* (pp. 197-221). Newbury Park, CA: Sage.

Relationships Among Older Women Living in a Nursing Home

Bethel Ann Powers, RN, PhD

SUMMARY. Literature suggests that women's skills in establishing close ties with other women help sustain them in old age by giving them a sense of control over their lives. This paper questions how such a notion may apply to women in a nursing home setting and contrasts women's experiences with those of men. It is a reanalysis of data from a previously reported study of institutionalized elders' social networks, this time with a specific focus on women residents' relationships with one another. Here, I consider the role of negative interaction in personal relationships, the meaning of intimacy and reciprocity in the nursing home context, and issues of age and gender. The final section, implications for practice and future research, includes a discussion of the opportunities for and constraints on relationship formation. *[Article copies available from The Haworth Document Delivery Service: 1-800-342-9678. E-mail address: getinfo@haworth.com]*

... women ... continue increasingly to outlive men, and to maintain and renew ties of intimacy that keep them in control of their later lives much longer than men ... females tend to establish closer, more intense ties with a smaller number of friends. Friendships between females have been found to be "emotionally richer" than

---

Bethel Ann Powers is Associate Professor, University of Rochester School of Nursing, Rochester, NY 14642.

[Haworth co-indexing entry note]: "Relationships Among Older Women Living in a Nursing Home." Powers, Bethel Ann. Co-published simultaneously in the *Journal of Women & Aging* (The Haworth Press, Inc.) Vol. 8, Nos. 3/4, 1996, pp. 179-198; and: *Relationships Between Women in Later Life* (ed: Karen A. Roberto) The Haworth Press, Inc., 1996, pp. 179-198; and: *Relationships Between Women in Later Life* (ed: Karen A. Roberto) Harrington Park Press, an imprint of The Haworth Press, Inc., 1996, pp. 179-198. [Single or multiple copies of this article are available from the Haworth Document Delivery Service: 1-800-342-9678, 9:00 a.m. - 5:00 p.m. (EST). E-mail address: getinfo@haworth.com]

friendships between males . . . the ability to share feelings, the
presence of a confidant . . . seems to constitute the essential intimacy.
(Friedan, 1993, pp. 261-262)

The literature on friendships in later life suggests that as people age
numbers of friends decline and there is less motivation to initiate new
relationships (Allan & Adams, 1989; Roberto, 1989). While factors
associated with aging such as decreasing mobility and increasing frailty
may account for less socialization, researchers have identified gender as
having the most significant influence on the shaping of friendship patterns
(Adams & Blieszner, 1989; Bell, 1981; Johnson & Troll, 1994). Women
have more social skills, more readily join activities that provide opportunities for socializing and meeting new people, are more expressive and
gregarious, and form deeper emotional attachments than men (Bell, 1981;
Friedan, 1993; Rubinstein, 1986).

Personality and previous lifestyles make a difference in the ways
women approach late life relationships. Physical condition and social circumstances also are factors that influence the degree to which women may
exercise abilities to extend and receive care and support and to initiate
personal exchanges in relationships with one another. In this paper, institutionalization is the common social circumstance within which frail elders
meet and interact.

The study setting was a 212-bed urban health-related facility, housed
within a county-operated long-term care institution that also provides acute
and skilled levels of care. The interior of this architecturally imposing
cluster of connected buildings was austere, with the long tiled corridors and
high ceilings reminiscent of its historical origins as county home and conva-
lescent hospital. Two- and four-bed semi-private rooms had replaced some
large patient wards of earlier decades and there were communal bathrooms
on each floor. Spacious enclosed porches and other common areas provided
a variety of places to sit, visit, and/or watch television. Each floor had a
small dining area. However, most residents took their meals in a large
dining room on the first floor. The more oriented and able-bodied residents
moved more freely about the hospital and grounds. They often guided or
pushed the wheelchairs of less capable residents to and from meals and
activities. Furnishings were sparse with an eclectic mix of hospital-issue
beds, chairs, bureaus, and lockers with residents' personal effects that demonstrated scattered attempts to introduce a sense of homeliness to the predominant public institutional ambience of the place.

In contrast to one all-male and one all-female floor, two floors in the
health-related facility accommodated women at one end and men at the
other end of the hallway. Common areas separated the two ends, but

division sometimes was arbitrary with instances where the need to place more men or more women infringed on territorial imperatives. The presence of the opposite sex next door disturbed the women more so than the men; but, neither women's nor men's living spaces were spared the regular corridor traffic that occurred when residents from all floors assembled on different porches for various activities (e.g., clubs, Bible study, parties, religious services). This co-mingling at meals and activities both on and off different floors where residents lived increased their opportunities to broaden personal contacts and make acquaintances with others throughout the facility. The social aspects of this nursing home culture were the focus of the research.

After a brief review of the overall study, I will expand on themes drawn from field observations and women's responses regarding themselves and the other women with whom they lived. Following these thematic descriptions I will present a brief contrasting of women's and men's social networks. I then reflect on Friedan's assertion about the skills that sustain women in old age in light of what the research suggests with regard to negative interaction, intimacy and reciprocity, and issues of age and gender. In the final section, I highlight the studies findings with respect to practice issues and future research needs.

THE OVERALL STUDY

Participants

The following description of relationships among older institutionalized women comes from a study of the social networks of 69 elderly male ($n = 32$) and female ($n = 37$) residents of the health-related facility. Nursing staff helped identify persons who could participate in the research. Inclusion criteria required residents to be at least 55 years old and able to give reasonable and consistent responses to interview questions. They needed to be oriented to person and place, with memory intact enough to describe socialization patterns as structured by the interview. Ages of participants ranged from 55 to 95 years, with a mean age of 73. Many were frail with multiple chronic illnesses and physical limitations. None could completely care for themselves. However, to remain in a less acute setting required them to perform some self-care and be ambulatory or mobile with the aid of a wheelchair. The data subset on women and their relationships with other women within the resident-resident interactional sector is the focus of this report. (For findings related to issues of social support, self-perceived health, and relationships within different interactional sectors of networks see Powers, 1988a, 1988b, 1991, 1992, 1995).

The Interview

I used a network profile interview guide designed to elicit both objective and subjective measures of social interaction (Sokolovsky, 1980) to gather data on all direct contacts that residents had with people inside and outside the institution. The profile involved four sectors of interaction: resident-resident, resident-staff, resident-kin, and resident-outside friend or acquaintance. In two or more tape-recorded sessions of about two hours each, I elicited information from each resident about their lives pre- and post-institutionalization and characteristics of contacts within each sector; when, where, how, and how often contact took place; the sorts of things people talked about and did for one another; and which network members knew and interacted with other network members. Only after obtaining the extent and behavioral aspects of the network were questions asked about the subjective importance of network ties. Consequently, the networks were not limited to subjectively important people or friends.

While elicitation of network data was the primary focus in the taped sessions, a conversational interviewing style facilitated collection of other kinds of information about participants' daily routines, reactions to institutional life, and their general perceptions of how they were getting along. Field notes of additional conversations and observations also were kept.

Analysis of network data involved description and comparison on an item-by-item basis of (a) interactional characteristics of networks (i.e., interactional content, frequency and intensity of interactions; multiplexity—whether the tie provided one or more types of resource; and directionality—whether the resources tended to flow only in one direction) and (b) structural characteristics of networks (i.e., size, clustering and interconnectedness of network members).

Network Typology

Four types of networks were identified that differed in terms of size, clustering of ties, interconnectedness, and interactional characteristics:

1. *Institution-centered networks* were small with proportionally fewer outside as opposed to intrainstitutional contacts. Ties often were simple and of low intensity. Self-proclaimed "loners" developed their own routines that brought them into contact with individuals

who could meet needs for passing time or supplying tangible goods and services with a minimal amount of emotional involvement. High value was placed on self-reliance accompanied by resistance to bureaucratic control. In contrast, those in the group who were isolated due to loss of a highly supportive outside person were more apt to turn to staff as a source of dependent support and emotional attachment.

2. *Small-cluster networks* were variants of institution-centered networks that contained small close-knit cliques of residents who regularly spent time together and shared confidences with one another.

3. *Kin-centered networks* were those in which residents had an average of four relatives who visited and talked with them on a weekly or monthly basis. Emotional ties to families made it difficult for some individuals to accept institutional relationships or activities.

4. *Balanced networks* were the largest and demonstrated greater interconnectedness. A wide range of contacts across the different sectors of resident, staff, kin, and outside friend or acquaintance facilitated the flow of communication and support.

THE FINDINGS

Institutionalization introduces people to a life lived in the company of strangers, who may or may not become less strange and more friend-like over time. For most individuals it is an adjustment that involves weighing possibilities while sorting out positives and negatives in a new social arena where there is a noticeable reduction in the opportunities for control over one's life and choice of one's companions. Examination of interview transcripts and field notes revealed that elderly institutionalized women in this sample established interpersonal ties with one another that provided a basis for supportive exchange and the sharing of thoughts and feelings. However, these ties varied in terms of emotional intensity and reciprocity. Data associated with themes of resisting and welcoming relationships with strangers are presented below. The intent is to give a broad overview of what women's movements away from and toward relationships looked like without imposing a strict dichotomy (since all of the women resisted some and welcomed other relationships with fellow residents to a greater or lesser extent). Examples of women's views and experiences are drawn from the different network configurations as previously described. Quotes are coded by case number and age of participant.

Resisting Relationships. Overall, women in institution-centered, small cluster, and kin-centered networks were most likely to limit relationships or to engage superficially with other residents. For example, one participant with an institution-centered network had a set routine that involved contact with a variety of residents at meals and activities. While responsive in groups and accepting of casual conversation, she did not initiate interaction or sustain personal relationships. She claimed difficulty in remembering people and names. When not engaged in a structured activity, she usually could be found sitting alone and removed from others in a chair by the elevator. The following quotation reflects that, although she was not totally isolated, relationships with others were largely impersonal, and she tended to withdraw when left to her own devices.

> #45/75: I can't remember their [other residents'] names. They tell me, but I forget. I can't remember her [roommate's] name either . . . I speak to her [but] I don't ask her to do anything for me. I do for myself . . . I eat at the table with the people. I say "Hi" [and] when I get my food I go . . . I like bingo very much. Any kind of games I like . . . all kinds of movies . . . [and] TV . . . I will talk to anybody that wants to talk to me [but] I'd rather be just like I am–quiet and by myself.

Another participant with a small cluster network excluded other residents by limiting her relationships to two close companions. She remained strongly dependent on these residents for motherly care (from Jane)[1] and sisterly guidance (from Mary) while resisting the attentions of others.

> #19/76: Jane [roommate] helps me get dressed [and] puts me to bed. I'm her little girl . . . I go for walks with Mary. I like to visit the sick people and encourage them.

Some residents explained that their resistance to relationships with others was based on fear and a need to avoid upsetting behavior, for example:

> #55/55 (kin-centered network): I'm scared of 'em . . . You got so much . . . ya gotta deal with so much. And it's disturbing to your rest.

Others described their reticence to form relationships as a feature of their personalities. Two additional examples provided by women with kin-centered networks follow.

---

1. All names used here are fictitious.

#27/95: I'm a peculiar person, which is not to say I'm distant or anything, but I don't jump into acquaintances. I get along with 'em and as long as I can get along with 'em that's all that's necessary. I'm not an inquisitive person . . . I don't want you to open the book and tell me your life's history . . . just friendly.

#47/74: I get along with everybody but I ain't got no special friends. You know, a lot of women, they run with a bunch, but I always went by myself.

Both women invested energy primarily on relationships with family and long-time friends outside of the institution. Every day, participant #27 visited her son, who himself was a resident housed on a different unit in the same nursing home. She also spoke longingly about her "very good" neighbor: "They were all good, but she was close. I used to go over every day and talk to her. She sent me cards. I think she misses me." She claimed that her roommate was the only resident whom she really knew, and she was pleased about the willingness of the roommate's daughters to run errands for her and their kindness in asking if she needed anything when they came to see their mother.

Participant #47 focused her attention on frequent visits from her sister, and generally sat alone or moved about to meals and activities unaccompanied. However, when she went to church, she escorted one of her roommates: " . . . and lots of times I gotta help her put her clothes on, you know. I help as much as I can."

Physical proximity of roommates created opportunities for simple companionship and helpful exchanges, though perfect companions and true reciprocity often were difficult to attain. For example, participant #3 (kin-centered network) recalled previous roommates who had been better conversationalists than her current roommate, but relocation and differences over keeping windows open or shut had caused them to part. The following quotation suggests that her ideal companion would provide diversion between visits from family and periods of self-imposed solitude by being more sociable without invading her privacy. Not having to argue about the open window plus access to a television partially compensated for less than ideal companionship.

#3/88: I used to get a good conversation outa her [former roommate]. This roommate don't talk much. I don't know if she don't want to or why I don't know. But she's nice to me. I'd like her to talk more, as long as she don't want to know all my business or something like that. I don't care. She's good to be with anyway and she don't mind me watching her television.

Participant #53 (kin-centered network) thought private rooms would be preferable so that residents would not disturb one another as they went about their routines or entertained visitors. There was little dialogue or mutual assistance between herself and her roommate. However, she expressed a willingness, as shown in the following quotation, to extend aid within the limits of her ability to do so.

> #53/84: The woman that lives in the other part there [roommate] . . . I think she may be older than I am. She was trying to take that one thing [walker] and pull it along beside [her wheelchair], and I said, "I'm going down that way. Want me to carry that for ya?" And she didn't say "no" so I carried that right behind her 'til she told me. She thanked me for it. I don't mind doing things like that, but I can't do too much.

The women in the above examples, while not totally resistant to or rejecting of social interaction, were selective and cautious in forming relationships, especially of a close or intimate sort. They frequently opted for the minimum personal investment possible through more superficial interactions.

The seven women (19% of the women in the sample) with institution-centered networks were "loners" whose pre-institutional lives had provided limited opportunities for social interaction. Some received occasional visits from kin or former neighbors, but the greater reliance was on intrainstitutional contacts. They frequently voiced pride in their abilities to be independent and, sometimes, a desire to keep busy or be useful. For example, participant #14 was very interested in anyone she thought she could "help," often to the dismay of staff who interpreted her helping ways as interferences with their care of or plans for other residents. In her case, she thought of helping others not in terms of friendship and intimacy, which she resisted, but in terms of "having a job" or a purpose that helped her reassert some independence and prevented her from dwelling on her own unhappiness at being in a nursing home.

> #14/75: It's important to me to help anybody I can. After all, here I am down here just living off the land as it were, and I'm not used to that. I'm quite interested in that woman [adjoining table] at present. She's paralyzed all down one side [and] I felt the girls [staff] weren't taking much consideration of her difficulty. I've helped her some

because it's just my nature to want to help people, but [staff] don't like me coming over, so I don't dare go up 'cept at night . . . I talk to the new lady too, and she tells me her troubles; but I don't care to become real intimate.

For the two women (5% of the women in the sample) with small-cluster networks, interactions with multiple people in the institutional environment were buffered and possible overloading reduced by their concentration on one or two other women exclusively. For example, Lila (participant #44) was completely absorbed in caring for Maybert, a roommate with Alzheimer's Disease. Lila was unsteady and quite forgetful, but she seemed able to give some direction to Maybert. They attended mass regularly as well as on- and off-unit activities. Lila would sometimes decline invitations to activities she might have enjoyed because Maybert was not interested in attending. Maybert got upset if she could not find her roommate or if Lila was not close by. When Lila was not feeling well, Maybert would quietly sit beside her waiting for her to feel better. The two were constantly in each other's company, to the exclusion of all others.

> #44/67: I don't see anybody else . . . just Maybert. We live in the same room, and sleep here . . . We talk a lot together . . . We go to meals together too. She's a good girl–Maybert . . . a very nice lady.

Thirteen women (35% of the women in the sample) with kin-centered networks focused on family relationships to the exclusion of most other residents. For example, participant #13 identified residents in her network with whom she interacted, but she said she had very little to do with them.

> #13/76: Not as yet, honey. [No residents as friends.] I have to know a person a while before I would [call him/her a friend].

She claimed her children and brother, whom she saw regularly, as her closest friends and confidants.

The 15 women (41% of the women in the sample) with balanced networks were the least resistant to forming and maintaining ties with other residents. They differed in this respect from the foregoing examples of women with other network configurations. However, they also actively resisted relationships that caused them distress. For example, residents with good interpersonal skills and reasoning abilities understood their value to staff who might view them as helpful resources to their less capable peers. These pairings, however, sometimes did not work out because of the emotional drain on the more intact individual, as explained by participant #20:

> #20/58: I did have problems having a roommate I couldn't handle. It took me six months to get rid of her . . . I tried to help her, but I couldn't, and this all was building up inside of me . . . I think that they [staff] thought that I was sympathetic enough that I could handle it, but it didn't work out.

Many women also commented on the prevalence of gossip and how important it was to protect one's privacy by actively avoiding individuals identified as the worst offenders. For example, participant #21 described how some residents got "too personal" in their conversations or sought to overhear what others were saying so that they could continue to feed the gossip circles.

> #21/74: Susie . . . she's back where the telephone is. When she hears the phone ring, she comes out and listens to what the people are saying . . . I just leave her alone. I don't want too many friends that way . . . I'm making friends with the new old ladies that come in. Some of them [other residents], as I told you, are not inquisitive, they're ignorantly nosy, and I keep away from them.

Welcoming Relationships. In general, the women with balanced networks were less wary and more welcoming of relationships with other residents. They tended to be more socially active and willing to introduce themselves and initiate conversation. Some claimed to be naturally gregarious, but they all knew whom they wished to avoid; and, like women with other network configurations, they were selective in choosing close friends. In some cases the women described their close friends as confidants. For example, participant #63 identified as an intimate friend a woman with whom she regularly exchanged local gossip.

> #63/59: Catherine . . . She and I are intimate friends. She tells me everything that is to be told. She passes it on to me . . . She tells me [and] I know what happened to this one and that one.

Participant #56 spoke of concerns that she shared with a trusted friend, including an aggressive act by a resident and the death of another that had upset her.

> #56/71: Connie [is a confidant] . . . If you got a problem, go to her and she'll straighten you out on your thinking. Connie is right on the ball, and she gives good advice. When I have a problem around here, I tell Connie and she knows just what to do about it.

Participant #20 identified as her confidant a resident whom she found especially trustworthy.

> #20/58: Margaret is about the only one that I can talk to about anything . . . We're close . . . I can talk to her and I do the same for her. There's a few you wouldn't dare tell [anything] because they'd blab it all over.

Although the women viewed having close friends in whom they could confide as important, few women across networks claimed to have such intimate ties with other residents. They were more likely to identify family, outside friends, or institution staff as confidants. The close ties with other residents that they described revolved less around personal issues and more around daily shared experiences (Powers, 1991).

Some examples from balanced networks of what participants identified as "close friend" relationships included ones in which women ministered to others and relationships where the participant primarily was a recipient of care and support. For example, participant #1 regularly sought out residents whom she believed were more afflicted than herself. But she had a special affection for one woman whom she described as a close friend whom she had been visiting in her room on another unit of the nursing home for seven years.

> #1/78: When I first knew her . . . she'd lost one leg and she declared she'd never let them amputate the other one, but she had to, and then two years or so ago she had a stroke and can't talk. So when I visit her, I have to do all the talking. And she understands quite well. I gave her a book a friend gave to me. It has beautiful pictures . . . Usually when I go there, I pray with her.

Participant #63 sought out a former roommate, whom she described as a close friend, for help and companionship soon after moving to another room.

> #63/59: Well, she was hard of hearing and older (79 years). She has a daughter about my age. And, she had a TV, so of course I couldn't play my radio or TV. I couldn't hear it . . . We get along now. It's very nice. I take my sewing over to her, and she does my sewing; and she makes a snack, and we have peanut butter and jelly sandwiches. We both love peanut butter.

Participant #42 and #43 identified as close friends other women they could trust to aid and assist them. For example, staff encouraged residents to be as independent as possible. However, residents, as in the case of participant #42, sometimes interpreted this as lack of caring and sought sympathy from other residents in the form of personal assistance.

> #42/67: When I'm in the wheelchair . . . when they get the shoes and things ready for me . . . Martha will help me dress because the aides won't and I'm unable to do it alone.

Staff also discouraged residents from paying other residents for favors and services, as related by participant #43, who nonetheless found it important to have a dependable person to rely on for favors and services.

> #43/63: Peggy helps me out when the nurses don't know it . . . [For example] if she pushes me [in the wheelchair] they holler at her to quit . . . but she does take and wheel me . . . and if I want anything done, I ask her . . . I was told not to give her any money at all. I was giving her a little just to help her along . . . Now I keep saying I ain't got it, but I have. For Christmas I went shopping and bought her all she asked for [because] you ask her for something and she's right there. She's very good help . . . She never says "No."

The residents considered their close friends to be more than casual acquaintances. They were people one could seek out and comfortably spend time; ask for or exchange favors; and be more revealing of oneself. Women would make an effort to maintain such ties when changes in circumstances occurred. For example, participant #14 (institution-centered network) strove to continue a companionable relationship with a woman with whom she used to walk daily about the institution and the institution grounds. When the friend became incapacitated, she instituted a morning ritual that involved sharing food and feeding the birds together. She explained this relationship as an exception to her usual resistant stance toward close ties with others.

> #14/75: [Regarding her friend]: I don't make friends that easily . . . I'm kinda standoffish. Many people are just people to me rather than friends. Friends do something special, and friends are people you can do something for. I see Ethel [resident moved to another unit because of a broken hip] every morning . . . [Before], I used to go to her room and she used to come to mine and want me to go someplace with her, even when I didn't want to go too bad, [but] I went . . . I take food from the cafeteria, and I feed the birds in her room [on the window sill] too; I like to feed the birdies.

Overall, friendship was not a unitary concept among these residents. There were differences and similarities in the ways that women with particular network experiences resisted and welcomed relationships with one another (and male residents on occasion). Definitions of friendship varied as did patterns of resource exchange. Common types of resources exchanged by the residents included tangible goods (e.g., food, cigarettes, reading material, small money loans), services (e.g., sewing, mending, shopping and errands), personal assistance (e.g., with dressing or mobilization), advice and guidance, information (e.g., gossip), and companionship and visiting. However, the give and take in relationships was often less symmetrical than commonly associated with norms of reciprocity.

Women who claimed other residents as close friends typically maintained no more than a few of these relationships. However, there could be any number of network members from the resident sector who were simply "friends" because the women perceived them as pleasant, agreeable persons. Women also pointed out members of their networks who were "not friends" because of their annoying or upsetting behavior. Their perceptions of friends versus non-friends were formed based on observation and through regular interaction in settings that included each other's rooms, the dining hall, common areas such as porches or lounges, or the institution grounds. Opportunities to interact with "friends" varied. For example, dining companions interacted with great regularity, but the women might infrequently see a "friend" whose acquaintance they made at a less than regular activity, particularly if residing on a different nursing home unit. Women did not always distinguish between ordinary friends and acquaintances. Consequently, a summarization of "friends," as distinguished from "non-friends," seemed to represent what they may have viewed as the widest range of acceptable friendly or friend-like individuals available to them at the time. Levels of emotional intensity, even with "close friends," were less than residents attached to preinstitutional friendships. Nevertheless, women were very positive about good friendship ties with (and successful avoidances of) various ones of their peers in this nursing home setting.

Women's and Men's Social Networks

There were no major differences between women and men based on demographics such as age, health status, or length of institutionalization. There were differences, however, in predominant network type. Most men in this sample (20 participants, 62.5% of the sample) had institution-centered networks in contrast to most of the women who had balanced networks (15 participants, 41% of the sample) or kin-centered (13 participants, 35% of the sample). Although the men initially claimed to have no friends, it became clear that they also distinguished between a hierarchy of relationships with other residents that included (Powers, 1991):

1. Acquaintances: people you recognize and greet on occasion, but who are known casually and not seen every day.
2. "Buddies": more than casual acquaintances–people you "chum around with" and with whom you may exchange favors.
3. Friends: people upon whom one can rely for help and in whom one can confide.

Men's relationships were low in intensity and often superficial with few reported intrainstitutional friendships. However, relationships were reportedly satisfactory in terms of companionship and established routines of sharing meals, attending activities, or sitting quietly together. In comparison, the women in kin-centered and balanced networks had more social contacts and closer, more intense interaction with network members. In most of the cases, patterns of socialization seemed consistent with described preinstitutional lifestyles for men who claimed to be "loners" and for women who spoke of keeping busy with family duties and/or an active social life. However, as both men and women had a diminishing number of personal ties with people outside the institution, maintenance of socialization patterns relied increasingly on incorporating fellow residents into personal networks. Participants emphasized that relationships with other residents identified as friends and companions were qualitatively different from preinstitutional ties in terms of level of intimacy and ability to support the reliving of experiences and shared memories. They spoke with feeling and emotion of the loneliness of lost friendships and their inability to replace these types of bonds.

Men also resisted and welcomed relationships with other residents. They tended to be more verbally and physically aggressive than women in warding off unwanted contacts with others in the environment, and expressed fewer concerns about those with whom they interacted. However, men did care for and offer practical assistance to one another. Men with small cluster networks (3 participants, 9% of the men in the sample) and with balanced networks (4 participants, 12.5% of the men in the sample) provided the best examples of caring for and interest in others, for example:

> #9/94: (small cluster network) Frank and I kinda chum together . . . We visit in each other's rooms and eat together . . . He pushes my chair and we go off . . . have a beer . . . [visit] with the guys.

#69/73: (balanced network) I devote my time to Ken because he needs a roommate who'll give him some attention . . . I don't want to make him feel as though he's left out because he can't speak.

Men with institution-centered networks (20 participants, 62.5% of the men in the sample) and with kin-centered networks (5 participants, 16% of the men in the sample) were less interested in and patient with one another and more focused on themselves and their own needs, for example:

#5/73: (institution-centered network) I sit around with them and listen to their barking, and when I get tired, I go to bed . . . Bob is the only one I talk to . . . and he's a little wacky too . . . [Of] course, it took me a while to figure him out, but I made it.

#70/77: (kin-centered network) Quiet is the way I like it . . . guys walking back and forth and yelling and screaming at each other . . . I call my kids and friends so I have someone to talk to.

Reflection on the data produces an impression that the majority of men approached peer relationships differently than the majority of women. The evidence suggests that differences in their network configuration best explain these differences. More men in this study used limited network resources in superficial and self-interested ways in contrast to most of the women whose network experiences were richer and more complex. However, the differences between men and women within network type were less pronounced than those across network type comparisons.

CONCLUSIONS

I return to Friedan's (1993) earlier quoted assertion that women's skills in maintaining and renewing ties of intimacy through confidant relationships with other women help to sustain them in old age by giving them a sense of control over their lives. How does this notion apply to the women in the sample? What does the nursing home experience present in terms of opportunities for and constraints on formation of close friendships? And, what can be said about the women's experiences in contrast to those of the men in this study? The following discussions consider the role of negative interaction in personal relationships, the meaning of intimacy and reciprocity in the nursing home context, and issues of age and gender.

Negative Interaction

Generally, personal social networks included people perceived as supportive and may even be considered upsetting to individuals. In institutions such as nursing homes, the likelihood of having unwanted network members increases since multiple contacts and interactions with others are difficult to avoid. However, the women in this study often were successful in establishing limits and warding off negative interactions by resisting and evading relationships beyond their tolerance.

Krause (1995) has suggested that negative interactions play a larger role in determining people's satisfaction with social support than the actual amount of assistance and support received.

> Instead of arising from the helpful behaviors, the benefits of associating with others may attribute to the ability of social network members to stave off or avert negative interaction. This alternate view [of social support] suggests that those who develop interventions to bolster natural support systems may need to reconceptualize the basic thrust of their programs. Rather than attempting to encourage supportive behavior, these practitioners may want to focus on eradicating negative or upsetting interaction. (Krause, 1995, p. P59)

Protecting oneself from unwanted interaction with others involves judgment, self-knowledge, and some social abilities. When the environment does not make it easy to walk away, people need to consider how to distance themselves. The examples provided in this paper of women engaged in resisting and welcoming relationships with other women suggest thoughtfulness about initiating and shaping relationships. Women knew their own tolerance and what they wished to avoid (overextending themselves, invasion of privacy, overdependence on others beyond whatever support they could give), and they questioned what becoming involved with others meant to them personally (increased self-esteem through being useful and valued; companionship; information and advice; tangible goods; and services). They distanced themselves from unwanted interactions by "getting along with people" while holding them at a distance, refusing to speak to or involve themselves with certain others, focusing their energy on selected relationships, and appealing for assistance in specific situations, such as a request for a room change. In comparison with most men, whose networks and personal interactions were less complex, women seemed generally quicker to analyze and express various opinions about the nature of their relationships and slower to give up on one another in the sense of being more prone to offer care and assistance. In setting limits and avoiding negative relationships women tended to be more communicative and less confrontational than men.

Intimacy and Reciprocity

Both men and women emphasized that intimate relationships with fellow residents were different from those that they had enjoyed with friends from preinstitutional days. They believed it was not possible to recapture the deep familiarities of past friendships nurtured by trustful sharing of thoughts and feelings. They expressed reluctance to reveal much of a personal nature to fellow residents with whom they felt they had less in common. While they saw self-revelation as something to avoid for the sake of preserving privacy, trustworthiness remained an important issue in the cultivation of new friendships. Women, more often than men, identified other same-sex residents as close or intimate friends. They trusted intimate friends to understand their perspective, to provide information about what was happening in the social environment, and to be discreet. However, they did not think of them as confidants, people with whom one would share information of a personal nature.

Reliability, in addition to trustworthiness, was another quality of close friends. The residents established that they could count upon certain people to provide support through resource exchange. However, reciprocity, in the sense of an even balanced exchange, was not characteristic of relationships where one person might seem to be the giver and another the recipient of tangible aid and assistance. Beyond the stated pleasures of giving and receiving, the less tangible and more expressive aspects of friendship (i.e., spending time together, talking, and visiting) can serve as equalizers in this type of uneven exchange. Companionship of many sorts was a valuable commodity in this social environment.

Sometimes women would identify more casual acquaintances as friends. This is consistent with findings of Johnson and Troll (1994) in their research on late-life friendships. They suggest that, in response to constraints on friendship formation, individuals may redefine friendship norms and content, for example, by extending the definition of "friend" to include more casual acquaintances or by lowering their expectations for intimacy or shared interests as a necessary part of the relationship. Thus, they may "cast a wider net" in exchange for "relationships of less intimacy, shallow communication, and less commitment" (Johnson & Troll, 1994, p. 85). Within the social confines of the institution, being satisfied with less in a relationship increased the participants' opportunities to make new friends and have more of a social life.

Age and Gender

There is no uniform way in which women's relationships evolve in the nursing home setting. In this research, women with different network experiences were almost resistant to exploring the possibilities of forming relationships with other residents. Differences between women and men also seemed most related to network type. Most of the men had less rich and complex networks than many women in the study. More of the men had a history of being "loners" and, although some women also fit that category, others described themselves as socially active or gregarious people. Thus, the ability of women to augment friendship relationships with intrainstitutional ties seemed, in part, determined by their personality and preinstitutional lifestyle. This observation is consistent with those of others who have studied late-life friendship patterns in different settings (Johnson & Troll, 1994). However, the role that gender may play remains open for further study. Johnson and Troll (1994) observed that " . . . differences in life style between younger men and women that contribute to gender differences in friendships are much less apparent in the life styles of the oldest old" (p. 85).

IMPLICATIONS FOR PRACTICE AND FUTURE RESEARCH

This research showed the diversity of institutionalized elders. Some residents' network interactions reflected a continuation of patterns from their earlier lives. Others had experienced previous network change through loss or through new opportunities for relationship formation. Although it is possible to describe nursing home life in terms of residents' shared experiences, in practice, it is the diversity of responses to the culture that we must consider. The network typology offers a way to conceptualize different ways in which individuals may adjust to nursing home life. It also invites appreciation of variety in individuals' actions and concerns without labeling particular network types as more or less functional or socially acceptable.

Assessing the support residents derive from network members is another practice concern. This research points out that we should not underestimate the importance of seemingly casual relationships among nursing home residents. It also calls attention to the negative side of network interaction that is especially noticeable in the confining atmosphere of institutional living. Regardless of network type, few residents in this research thought that they could get along with everyone. Helping individuals avoid unnecessary upset and deal with negative interactions requires tact, sensitivity, and ingenuity.

The data suggest that it is difficult for elderly institutionalized women to maintain and reconstitute the type of intimate ties that, according to Friedan (1993), keep women in control of their later lives longer compared to men. Yet, they still may exert some control through successful avoidance of negative interaction and formation of new relationships. Replacing deeper emotional attachments with less demanding ones may help fill the void caused by multiple losses and physical separation from their past lives. Ties with other residents supplement contacts with kin and outside friends who are more likely than others to serve as confidants. These findings suggest the need for further study and comparison of women's pre- and post-institutional friendship patterns. In addition, we can enhance our comparisons of women's experiences with those of men by paying more attention to male-oriented studies. Considering the experiences of particular age cohorts across the lifespan also should be a consideration in future research. Upcoming generations may have different viewpoints and concerns than those expressed by today's elders. In any case, improving care in nursing homes needs to involve ongoing study of how institutional culture may present the least challenge while best accommodating individuals' diverse social relationship needs.

REFERENCES

Adams, R. G. & Blieszner, R. (Eds.) (1989). *Older adult friendships*. Newbury Park, CA: Sage.

Allan, G. A. & Adams, R. G. (1989). Aging and the structure of friendships. In R. G. Adams & R. Blieszner (Eds.), *Older adult friendships* (pp. 45-64). Newbury Park, CA: Sage.

Bell, R. (1981). *Worlds of friendship*. Beverly Hills, CA: Sage.

Friedan, B. (1993). *The fountain of age*. New York: Simon & Schuster.

Johnson, C. L. & Troll, L. E. (1994). Constraints and facilitators to friendships in late late life. *The Gerontologist, 34*, 79-87.

Krause, N. (1995). Negative interaction and satisfaction with social support among older adults. *Journals of Gerontology: Psychological Sciences, 50*, P59-P73.

Powers, B. A. (1988a). Social networks, social support, and elderly institutionalized people. *Advances in Nursing Science, 10* (2), 40-58.

Powers, B. A. (1988b). Self-perceived health of elderly institutionalized people. *Journal of Cross-Cultural Gerontology, 3*, 299-321.

Powers, B. A. (1991). The meaning of nursing home friendships. *Advances in Nursing Science, 14* (2), 42-58.

Powers, B. A. (1992). The roles staff play in the social networks of elderly people. *Social Science & Medicine, 34*, 1335-1343.

Powers, B. A. (1995). From the inside out: The world of the institutionalized elderly. In J. N. Henderson & M. D. Vesperi (Eds.), *The culture of long term care: Nursing home ethnography* (pp. 179-196). Westport, CT: Bergin & Garvey.

Roberto, K. A. (1989). Exchange and equity in friendships. In R. Adams & R. Blieszner (Eds.), *Older adult friendships* (pp. 147-165). Newbury Park, CA: Sage.

Rubinstein, R. L. (1986). *Singular paths: Old men living alone.* New York: Columbia University Press.

Sokolovsky, J. (1980). Interactional dimensions of the aged: Social network mapping. In C. Fry & J. Keith (Eds.), *New methods for old age research* (pp. 75-100). Chicago: Center for Urban Policy.

Index

199

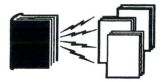

Haworth
DOCUMENT DELIVERY
SERVICE

This valuable service provides a single-article order form for any article from a Haworth journal.

- *Time Saving:* No running around from library to library to find a specific article.
- *Cost Effective:* All costs are kept down to a minimum.
- *Fast Delivery:* Choose from several options, including same-day FAX.
- *No Copyright Hassles:* You will be supplied by the original publisher.
- *Easy Payment:* Choose from several easy payment methods.

Open Accounts Welcome for . . .
- Library Interlibrary Loan Departments
- Library Network/Consortia Wishing to Provide Single-Article Services
- Indexing/Abstracting Services with Single Article Provision Services
- Document Provision Brokers and Freelance Information Service Providers

---

MAIL or *FAX* THIS ENTIRE ORDER FORM TO:

Haworth Document Delivery Service
The Haworth Press, Inc.
10 Alice Street
Binghamton, NY 13904-1580

or FAX: 1-800-895-0582
or CALL: 1-800-342-9678
9am-5pm EST

PLEASE SEND ME PHOTOCOPIES OF THE FOLLOWING SINGLE ARTICLES:

1) Journal Title: _____
    Vol/Issue/Year: _____ Starting & Ending Pages: _____
Article Title: _____

2) Journal Title: _____
    Vol/Issue/Year: _____ Starting & Ending Pages: _____
Article Title: _____

3) Journal Title: _____
    Vol/Issue/Year: _____ Starting & Ending Pages: _____
Article Title: _____

4) Journal Title: _____
    Vol/Issue/Year: _____ Starting & Ending Pages: _____
Article Title: _____

(See other side for Costs and Payment Information)

COSTS: Please figure your cost to order quality copies of an article.

1. Set-up charge per article: $8.00
         ($8.00 × number of separate articles)   _____

2. Photocopying charge for each article:
         1-10 pages: $1.00   _____

         11-19 pages: $3.00   _____

         20-29 pages: $5.00   _____

         30+ pages: $2.00/10 pages   _____

3. Flexicover (optional): $2.00/article   _____

4. Postage & Handling: US: $1.00 for the first article/
         $.50 each additional article   _____

         Federal Express: $25.00   _____

         Outside US: $2.00 for first article/
         $.50 each additional article_____

5. Same-day FAX service: $.35 per page   _____

                GRAND TOTAL: _____

METHOD OF PAYMENT: (please check one)

❏ Check enclosed   ❏ Please ship and bill. PO # _____
      (sorry we can ship and bill to bookstores only! All others must pre-pay)

❏ Charge to my credit card: ❏ Visa; ❏ MasterCard; ❏ Discover;
      ❏ American Express;

Account Number:_____ Expiration date:_____

Signature: ✗ _____

Name: _____ Institution: _____

Address: _____

_____

City: _____ State: _____ Zip:_____

Phone Number: _____ FAX Number: _____

MAIL or *FAX* THIS ENTIRE ORDER FORM TO:

Haworth Document Delivery Service | **or FAX:** 1-800-895-0582
The Haworth Press, Inc. | **or CALL:** 1-800-342-9678
10 Alice Street | 9am-5pm EST)
Binghamton, NY 13904-1580